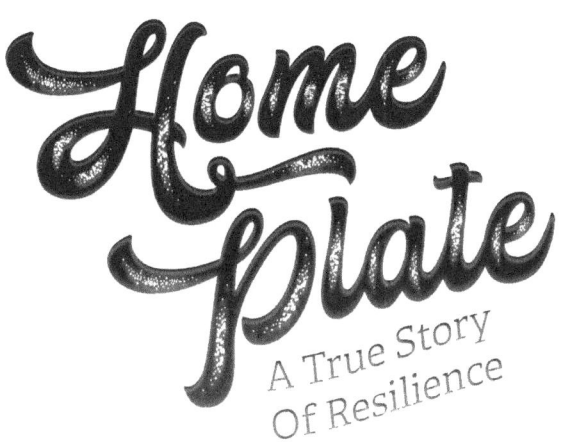

Home Plate
A True Story Of Resilience

BY STEPHANIE WALLS AND REMINGTON WALLS

All rights reserved. No part of this publication may be reproduced, distributed, or transmitted in any form or by any means, including photocopying, recording, or other electronic or mechanical methods, without the prior written permission of the publisher, except in the case of brief quotations embodied in critical reviews and certain other noncommercial uses permitted by copyright law.

Copyright © 2020 Stephanie Walls

TheHomePlateStory.com

ISBN: 978-1-7369904-9-0

Dedication

This book is dedicated to anyone experiencing a life-altering disease. It is our hope that this book might encourage you to continue pushing forward, looking up, and never settling for the limitations others put on you.

A special thanks to my husband Mike for his unwavering strength, my son Dalton for his sense of humor and endless chatter, my son Remington for his courage, and my mom for her positivity. To our family and friends (you know who you are), we've been blessed by you. Most importantly, thank you God for blessing us with the strength to stay the course.

—S<small>TEPHANIE</small> W<small>ALLS</small>

Home Plate

This book is dedicated to those who helped me get to where I am today, especially to my friends who accepted me for who I am and didn't treat me any differently. To the kids just like me and to others who are fighting different battles: Keep fighting and never give up.

A special thanks to my mom and dad, my brother Dalton, my closest friends, my trainer Larry, and my pastor Chris.

—REMINGTON WALLS

Contents

Dedication 3

Foreword 7

Part One 13

Chapter 1:
The First Signs 15

Chapter 2:
The Diagnosis 23

Chapter 3:
Life Changes 31

Chapter 4:
The New Normal 39

Part Two 55

Chapter 5:
Baseball and Art..57

Chapter 6:
School Days..69

Chapter 7:
Almost Quitting..77

Chapter 8:
Accepting Help..89

Chapter 9:
Helping Others..101

Chapter 10:
A Note from Dad..111

Chapter 11:
How to Truly Live...123

Chapter 12:
An Update from the Walls Family.....................133

Resources...145

About the Authors...149

Foreword

Dear Reader,

When you first meet Remington Walls, "rare" and "chronic illness" are not likely to be the first words that come to mind. Instead you see a young man who is confident, mature beyond his years, and who appears…well, healthy!

But for those who know Remington and know the journey he has been through with eosinophilic esophagitis, a few words that come to mind are resilient, remarkable, and unshakable.

Eosinophilic esophagitis (EoE) is a chronic, allergic inflammatory disease of the esophagus (the tube connecting the mouth to the stomach). It occurs when a type of white blood cell, the eosinophil, accumulates in the esophagus, causing injury and inflammation to the esophagus. This damage may make eating difficult or uncomfortable, potentially resulting in poor growth, chronic pain, and/or difficulty swallowing.

Symptoms may vary from one individual to the next.

Infants and toddlers often refuse their food or have trouble growing properly. School-age children may have recurring abdominal pain, trouble swallowing, or vomiting. Adolescents and adults most often experience difficult or painful swallowing. Their esophagus may narrow over time, increasing the potential for food to become stuck, which can result in a medical emergency. While the exact cause of EoE is not yet known, the general belief is that it's most often caused by an immune response to specific foods.

The Walls family are EoE pioneers. At the time Remington was diagnosed, far less was known about this condition and it took patients a very long time and multiple specialists before being diagnosed. Today, thanks to the hard work of researchers, organizations like APFED, clinicians, and patient advocates, there are consensus guidelines and a wealth of resources to help guide the recognition, diagnosis, and management of EoE.

While the road to diagnosis has greatly improved for families today, the diagnostic tools and therapeutic options have not. As of this writing, diagnosis can only be accomplished with esophageal biopsies that are obtained while the patient is under anesthesia – a procedure that is repeated often throughout the patients' lives to help monitor their condition and their response to therapy.

As of this writing, there is no FDA-approved therapy to treat EoE. The two main treatments utilized are medication used off-label (approved for other conditions, but not specifically for EoE) and diet management. Medications may include topical steroids (fluticasone or budesonide), swallowed from an asthma inhaler or mixture to control inflammation and suppress the eosinophils. Diet management includes removing known or suspected food triggers. For some patients, such as Remington, the dietary restrictions may be so severe, that nutrition must be obtained in full or in part by specialized formula. For some, a feeding tube may be needed.

Can you imagine what it must be like to be told that in order to treat your condition, you must give up all food and rely only on a specialized (and expensive!) formula for sustenance? Can you imagine if it were your child, and you had to explain to them why they couldn't eat like everyone else? Or the anxiety you would feel about sending them to school or to participate in social activities where food is inevitably present? Or having to restructure family holidays that traditionally involve food, like Thanksgiving?

It's no easy feat by any stretch of the imagination. The Walls family has accomplished this and so much more. They are a shining example of making the finest lemonade out of all of life's lemons. Rather than giving up, they shifted their focus from food to doing all they could to help others who found themselves in the same boat. They have worked tirelessly to support research initiatives, to advocate for the insurance coverage of medical foods such as the formulas prescribed to treat EoE, to raise awareness and educate the public about these conditions, and to help families learn that they too can live well with EoE. They have raised Remington to take EoE in stride and to find the work-around to challenges. They have taught him to take control over his disease, rather than allow the disease to control him. They have shown him how to advocate. They have taught him compassion and how to help others find their way, too.

The Walls family have been tried and true members of APFED's patient community for a very long time. I have had the pleasure of getting to know Stephanie over the years and she and I share a belief that things happen for a reason. I truly believe that her family was destined to share their "lemonade recipe" and their message of hope to families all over the globe. I have been honored to work with Stephanie on a number of initiatives. She has accomplished so much and I am grateful for all she has done in support of the EoE patient community.

On behalf of patients everywhere who live with eosinophil-associated diseases, thank you for taking the time and interest in reading Remington's story and learning about the challenges that so many of the people in our community face. If you or a loved one have an eosinophil-associated disease, I hope this story leaves you inspired, motivated, and empowered.

And to Remington: We will always be your biggest fans.

Mary Jo Strobel
Executive Director
The American Partnership for Eosinophilic Disorders

The American Partnership for Eosinophilic Disorders (APFED) is a 501c3 nonprofit organization founded in 2001. APFED's mission is to passionately embrace, support, and improve the lives of patients and families affected by eosinophil-associated diseases through education and awareness, research, support, and advocacy. Learn more at apfed.org.

Home Plate

Part One

*As told by Stephanie Walls with comments
from Remington.*

Chapter 1:

The First Signs

Remington: (Olde English); a man of many great things.

When we put that on our son's birth certificate, we had no idea how true that statement would eventually become. Remington was the name we chose for our second son. His older brother Dalton's name also had Olde English roots and we had thought we were simply choosing a similar type name. We wanted to choose a name that had the ending of "ton" just like his older brother's. Both were chosen from a Christian baby book of names and their meanings. However, we had no idea how important Remington's name would be or how it would come to be a rock we could all stand on when the days grew dark.

Almost from the second we brought Remington home from the hospital, we knew something was wrong with him. Every time he drank formula, he got sick. He would spit up repeatedly and barely held down anything. We changed his formula. No change.

Home Plate

Remington fussed, cried, and screamed more than Dalton, who was born five years earlier, ever had. At times, Dalton walked around the house with his fingers in his ears to block out the loud cries of his little brother.

Remington caught just about every type of germ. He continually had ear infections, high fevers, vomiting, and diarrhea, all of which kept him from gaining weight and growing like he should. Then came the colic. When he was two months old, he began screaming uncontrollably for hours on end and didn't stop for four more months. I remember putting Remington into his car seat and placing it on top of the running dryer, hoping the motion and white noise would calm him down. I sat on a bar stool next to the dryer and sang to him, staying there as long as I needed to, frustrated and at a loss for what to do to ease my baby's pain.

Nothing seemed to work. Not swaddling him, not holding him, not singing—nothing. Even after the colic stopped when he was six months old, he continued to have problems keeping the formula down and gaining weight. He fussed and cried and was so sleep-deprived that he had dark circles under his eyes. He looked at me with that pleading in his eyes that said: *there's something wrong with me, Mom. Fix it. Please.*

The First Signs

It killed us. Mike and I would stay up late into the night, researching, talking, and trying to figure out what was wrong with our youngest child. We prayed for answers, prayed for relief, and sometimes just prayed because we felt so lost.

We kept going back to the doctors. We tried everything, every test possible, including CT scans for tumors, injecting dyes to analyze him inside, etc. No one could tell us what the problem was or what was wrong with Remington. This went on for two long years—our baby crying and struggling to keep food down—and the doctors shaking their heads and saying they didn't have an answer.

Every parent dreams of their child's first birthday party. The baby in the high chair, a slice of birthday cake in front of him, and a mess of cake mushed on his face and clothes. Dalton had had that, and when Remington's first birthday came, we invited our relatives and sat him in the high chair—he played with his cake just like other children do, but after he ate some he began the requisite coughing and gagging episodes now routine when he ate.

By the age of two, with numerous doctors' visits behind us, Remington still wasn't getting better. He hated to eat anything. He choked, gagged, vomited,

Home Plate

fussed, had diarrhea, and cried constantly. Dinner time became a nightmare for all of us because every meal involved screaming and tantrums. Dalton was seven by then, chatty and amiable, but the fun, family mealtime we'd envisioned became a nightmare we dreaded. Our tempers grew short, and there were times when both of us had just had it with the screaming and the noise. We were so frustrated. Families are supposed to enjoy their new baby and build memories through birthday parties, and Friday night pizzas, and early morning pancakes . . . but we had none of that with Remington.

When yet another plate of food ended up on the floor, I headed into the pediatrician's office with my underweight, pained boy, and demanded answers. He recommended we see a gastroenterologist. Just from looking at him, she said she knew what the problem was. Acid Reflux.

She never scoped him or ran any kind of test. She just placed Remington on steroids along with a nebulizer to use twice a day. We were told to continue with his normal diet, which at that age was all the things regular kids like to eat—pasta, chicken nuggets, cereal, or fruit. All the foods other kids loved, Remington hated. He cried and screamed and refused them all. After three months on this new plan and several more doc-

The First Signs

tor's visits, we hadn't seen any changes in Remington. His eyes had become dark, sad puddles. His cheeks were hollowed. And worse, he rarely smiled.

At the time, we had no idea what that diagnosis would mean or how it would change not only our lives, but the lives of so many people around us.

Everything in our little boy was saying *help me*. We just didn't know how, and it broke our hearts.

> *There are photos of me as a baby, sitting in a high chair with spaghetti all over my face and hands, as well as the tray. My parents said that I loved spaghetti so much that when I would eat it, they would just have me sit in my diaper in the high chair because I would use both of my hands to shovel it in as fast as I could. They said I would get so messy that it was easier to have me eat half naked so they could give me a bath when I was done. None of us knew that what I loved most to eat in the world was also slowly killing me or that there would come a day when I would have to say goodbye to spaghetti and cereal and cookies—the foods other kids take for granted."*

19

Home Plate

The GI doctor kept saying, "Give it three more months." Eventually, we stopped going to her. Nothing was changing and Remington only seemed to get worse the older he got.

We were in an impossible situation. Mike and I aren't doctors, and when all the tests kept coming back negative we were as stumped as the medical professionals. Between caring for one busy boy and one miserable, crying toddler, we were exhausted. We blamed ourselves for not researching enough and not taking more control. We listened to the doctors because they had all those degrees on the wall and were supposed to be the experts.

We refused to give up. When Remington was three, we went back to the pediatrician again and told him that we needed a referral for another GI doctor. Going into that appointment, we were exhausted and pessimistic. No one had been able to help us or make a diagnosis.

This new doctor started talking about performing a scope on Remington, and a Ph test probe. That meant Rem staying the night in the hospital, but it was a test that might finally give us answers.

That scope did indeed give us a diagnosis and a name for what Remington was suffering. It was a start and a direction. At the time, we had no idea what that diagnosis would mean or how it would change not only our lives, but the lives of so many people around us.

Chapter 2:

The Diagnosis

Eosinophilic Esophagitis.

We stood in the waiting room listening to the doctor say those words, and a part of me knew this was it. This was the diagnosis we had been searching for all these years.

Eosinophilic Esophagitis is an inflammatory condition of the esophagus in which the wall of the esophagus becomes filled with large numbers of eosinophils, a type of white blood cell. These white blood cells are manufactured in the bone marrow and can create inflammation in the body, when high amounts of eosinophils are present. In EoE, a large number of eosinophils can accumulate in the esophagus, eventually stiffening this muscular tube so much, solid food can't pass to the stomach. It's diagnosed through an endoscopy and biopsy of the tissues of the esophagus.

Home Plate

That first scope showed that Remington had EoE in his upper esophagus. Mike and I were stunned by this news but grateful we finally had an answer. Not all doctors know about EoE, or how to diagnose it, so we were lucky that our path led to Dr. Thiru Arasu for correctly diagnosing Rem. Dr. Arasu told us he had recently read about EoE and later attended a conference where EoE had been discussed.

> *We were so lost, so scared, and we needed guidance from above.*

Inside the surgical suite, our little boy was still asleep, his arm curled around a stuffed Mickey Mouse who'd been fitted with his own surgical mask to make three-year-old Remington feel more at ease. He looked so small and fragile, too young to have such big words surrounding his life.

After Rem's scope, we were referred to an allergist in the Tampa Bay area who took Remington off of the six high-allergy foods: wheat, soy, eggs, milk, nuts, and shellfish. He was to continue eating everything else—beef, vegetables, fruits, rice, etc. However, Remington wasn't getting any better. He still vomited, gagged, choked, and had diarrhea. He was on the bottom of the growth analysis chart for children his age because he wasn't ingesting the proper nutrition.

The Diagnosis

His eyes still looked so pained, rimmed by dark circles, and his face was still so hollow. Six months after Remington's first scope we had him scoped again. This time, the eosinophils had spread to his lower esophagus.

If nothing was done, Remington would lose his ability to swallow anything at all.

We were devastated by the news. Out in the hall, Mike and I looked at each other, the same thought running through our minds—if we didn't figure this out, there was a possibility our child would be malnourished or worse, possibly die from malnutrition.

I got down on my knees and prayed. I begged and pleaded with God for my son's health. We were so lost, so scared, and we needed guidance from above. I whispered over and over, "Please, just give me a sign. What do we do? How do we save him?"

That afternoon, I spent hours educating myself on EoE. I researched doctors, treatments, hospitals, and eventually came across the Cincinnati Children's Hospital Medical Center. CCHMC had a research clinic for eosinophilic-related diseases. It was Sunday and the eosinophilic clinic office was closed, but I left them a desperate, pleading voicemail.

Monday morning, the clinic called me back. It was amazing just having someone to talk to who knew what I was experiencing. I felt as if God had answered my prayers, giving us a direction to follow and a destination that just might save our son.

We made an appointment to meet the doctors in October 2004. After yet another scope, the doctors confirmed Remington did have EoE in his lower and upper esophagus. Our doctor at CCHMC, Philip Putnam, recommended Remington be taken off all food and drink and replace it all with an elemental formula.

It took us a minute to absorb this information. No food or drink other than water, *literally*. No milkshakes, no chicken, no apples or grapes, or anything that the rest of us took for granted as part of our daily meals. The very things meant to nourish our bodies were destroying Remington's from the inside out. His body needed to heal, and the only way for that to happen was to avoid all the things hurting it.

Basically, the doctor explained, when Remington ate food, the eosinophils caused the tissue in his esophagus to deteriorate. We all have eosinophils, but Remington

The Diagnosis

had a higher concentration located in his esophagus. When food entered his body, the eosinophils attack the food as if it's an enemy and then continue attacking the tissue in his esophagus. For him, this is incredibly painful because his esophageal tissue becomes grooved and ridged, losing its elasticity. If nothing was done, Remington would lose his ability to swallow anything at all.

Children and adults suffering from EoE often need to have a feeding tube inserted to bypass the esophagus and be fed directly into the stomach because they aren't able to drink enough elemental formula and maintain proper nutrition. After we sat down with Remington and explained the diagnosis, we had to break this reality to our little boy. A feeding tube meant limiting his activities to keep it from dislodging, and Remington was adamant that he never wanted one because then he wouldn't be able to play baseball. We vowed to Remington that we would support him in this and do whatever we could to help him avoid a tube but that his health came first.

That day, all four of us—Mike, myself, Dalton, and Remington—left the hospital feeling numb and shell-shocked. We were silent the whole two-hour drive back to Columbus, which became our hub any time we had appointments at CCHMC. We were fortunate to have my cousin, Linda, and her husband, Collin, open their

Home Plate

home to us for each of our trips; yet another blessing from God.

When we got home, we sent the boys upstairs to take showers while Mike and I went out to the back deck. The world was perfect beyond the yard—blue sky, green trees, birds singing—but our world had just turned dark, and stormy, and scary. All those hours of talking and driving, both of us being strong in front of our sons and hiding our fear from Remington, fell apart once we were alone. Mike and I stood on that deck, clung to each other, and just cried and cried.

We called our families and filled them in on the news. Each time we recounted the details of Remington's disease, it hurt all over again. For hours that night, Mike and I talked about what to do, circling around our decisions like lost rats in a maze. Should we move from Florida to Ohio to be closer to the hospital? Should we sell the house? Change jobs? Pull Dalton out of school and uproot our boys? Or stay in Florida?

It was like we were plopped in the middle of a test without any research or review or tools to know which answer to choose. All we had was a diagnosis and a stack of information. Asleep upstairs, we had a four-year-old whose life had just dramatically and irrevocably changed.

I barely slept that night. I doubt Mike slept much either. In the morning, I sat at the kitchen table, holding the brochures the hospital had given us. At the bottom of the pile, I saw one from The American Partnership for Eosinophilic Disorders. The words *resources, support,* and *community* jumped out at me. As I picked up the phone to call them, I began to feel a little bit of hope for the first time since hearing the words *Eosinophilic Esophagitis.*

Chapter 3:

Life Changes

After the diagnosis, regular life changed dramatically, not just for us, but for Remington, too. When the doctors first said, "He can't eat any regular food or drink any regular drinks," I don't think it quite sank in until that first meal at home. The first one in a restaurant. Or the first birthday party. Those moments drove home the reality of Rem's diagnosis and what it meant to his life.

I sobbed a lot during the first couple of years after my diagnosis. I was only four and I didn't understand why I couldn't eat the same things as my brother or my friends. I thought of how unfair my life was and how I really wanted to have things like cookies and hamburgers. I could smell the food, see other people eat it, but it was, essentially, toxic to me if I ate it. But at four, you don't really understand that. All you hear is the word no. It took me a long time to come to terms with my EoE diagnosis.

Home Plate

> *When I cried, my dad would pick me up, sit me on his lap, and hug me tight. My brother, who was only nine, didn't know how to make me happy (and I don't think he totally understood everything either), so he'd stand there, trying to give me one of his favorite toys. Other times, Dalton would invite me into his room to color. We would lie on the floor with the books spread out, crayons in a circle on the carpet, and we'd color and just talk. Like normal kids. In those moments, I felt normal and I could forget about the next shake or the next meal, or the next birthday party. I could just be a kid."*

Periodically, Remington would undergo food trials to try one food at a time, testing whether he would react or if he could add that food back into his diet. If he started coughing and gagging or had any pain, he had to stop eating the food. He was so young, though, it was hard for him to tell us that he hurt. Besides, like all kids, he liked most foods and didn't want to give anything up, so sometimes he wouldn't tell us how the food made him feel.

We continued meeting his nutritional requirements with the elemental formula, but it was a tough adjustment for him. The formula's bitter aftertaste and the sheer volume Remington needed to drink every day to

Life Changes

keep up with the needs of his growing body was overwhelming.

Additionally, Remington met with an allergist to have patch and skin prick testing done. For those tests, he wore little "patches" of food on his back for several days. He'd return to the doctor's office several times to have the readings checked to determine if he was allergic to anything. On top of that, Remington underwent regular scopes so the doctor could see if Rem's esophagus showed signs of damage. Each time, he'd take a biopsy showing the eosinophil count and whether or not Rem still had active esophagitis. The scope pictures gave us a preliminary answer on the food trials and the biopsy was used for confirmation.

Imagine only being able to drink one thing for the rest of your life.

As time progressed, food trials became a grueling experience for Remington. Every food he tried, his body rejected. Nothing worked, and we always had to fall back on only consuming the elemental formula. We were all incredibly frustrated. Mike and I prayed constantly for answers for our little boy.

Home Plate

The entire situation was extremely difficult for us as parents, too. There were days when we couldn't see a positive ending to this situation. We were scared, lost, and felt alone, but our son was the one who suffered the most.

Imagine only being able to drink one thing for the rest of your life. To stand in the kitchen and smell food cooking or hear the sizzle of a steak on the grill and know you couldn't eat any of it. Rem struggled with seeing food or watching us eat. We began cooking outside on the grill and took turns eating—basically becoming closet eaters. Mike and I took turns and took a plate into our room and ate and Dalton ate with one of us. That way, one of us could help keep Remington entertained while the others were eating. We thought we were helping him—in reality, each we ate away from him caused us to be more and more dysfunctional as a family.

What used to be a nightly routine—sitting together as a family around the table, saying grace, and eating dinner while talking to one another and sharing our day—had become something we all avoided. We could see our family slowly unraveling at the seams because we weren't connecting. We were just passing each other, barely even saying hello to one another, because all of

Life Changes

our energy went to keeping Remington calm and distracted from food.

> *Remington's pain and depression went incredibly deep and was not something we could fix overnight.*

When Remington was five, he began having a temper tantrum one morning on the way to school. These had become a regular occurrence, as his frustration with his situation grew with every passing day. He began screaming about how his life wasn't fair and that he hated his life. Everything I tried to say only seemed to make it worse and he started screaming, "I wish I was dead!" at the top of his lungs.

The words shocked me. I pulled over and whispered a quick prayer, asking God what to do. What could I say to my son who was hurting so deeply? I unhooked my seat belt and dashed over to his side of the car to scoop him up and hug him fiercely. Rem sobbed in my arms—my little boy was far too young to be so broken, but there we were.

I couldn't take him to school like that. Frankly, I didn't even want to leave him. I knew he had reached the end of his rope, and so had we. This disease had taken our entire family hostage. I called in sick to work and then

Home Plate

called Mike. I told him I was calling the counselor immediately to get us in. He referred us to a psychiatrist, who got us in that day.

The psychiatrist confirmed that Remington was exhibiting signs of depression. He said that Remington was overstressed for such a young boy and that his mental well-being was in jeopardy. The psychiatrist explained to us that Remington didn't fully understand his situation and believed we were withholding food as punishment because of his disease.

The psychiatrist was firm with us, making it clear that a child Remington's age should know happiness and joy and not be wishing for death. Remington's pain and depression went incredibly deep and was not something we could fix overnight.

I have always found strength through prayer but in that moment, when my seven-year-old son was asking me if he was going to die, I found myself questioning God.

We were petrified. Mike and I realized we had a son whose pain was far worse than anything we had imagined. We felt so ashamed and humiliated that our son had reached such a place of

Life Changes

desperation. How could we as parents not see our child hurting? Not known that it had gotten this bad?

We had other moments over the years. One night, when I was tucking Remington into bed the night before we were leaving for yet another trip to the hospital. He looked up at me and asked, "Mom, am I going to die?" The words came out of nowhere. Horrified, I asked him why he'd ask such a thing. "Because I'm not getting any better."

I climbed up in bed next to him and wrapped my arms around him and said, "Remington, one day we all will die, but I don't believe that's any time soon." We talked about the importance of believing in God and I reminded him how courageous he'd been through it all. I also reminded him that it didn't mean he wasn't getting better just because he wasn't able to eat. I reassured him he *was* better; his body was healthier and he was growing. That was all that mattered. But most of all, I held him and loved him.

I have always found strength through prayer but in that moment, when my seven-year-old son was asking me if he was going to die, I found myself questioning God. Is it not enough that my son can't eat? Is it not enough that we're doing the best we can to accommodate all of these medical expenses to care for him? When I was alone, I tried to pray, but I found myself screaming at Him instead. "What do you want from me, God?"

And then, when I was finally quiet, I heard God answer, "I want you to trust Me." I realized that I was trying to control the situation. I was so focused on what I needed to do to fix my son that I had lost focus on what God wanted for the direction of our lives. From the day he was diagnosed, we told Remington that he was chosen to walk this path so that he could help others along the way. Until that moment, I hadn't really believed it myself. God was giving me a reminder that it would all be okay—we just needed to take it one day at a time. That night I read Romans 5: 3-4:

> *Not only so, but we also glory in our sufferings, because we know that suffering produces perseverance; perseverance, character; and character, hope. (NIV)*

From that day forward, HOPE became our family's word.

Chapter 4:

The New Normal

Throughout all of this, we still had another son who needed our attention and devotion. We were often so focused on Remington and his illness that we sometimes neglected our older boy, Dalton. When you have one sick child, though, it's hard not to give him all your attention and worry. Our lives revolved around the EoE at first—around food and formula, and trying to find the best course of action for Rem.

We were so far from a normal family that to be with friends around food was extremely difficult.

The four of us used to do so many activities together, like going to the zoo, to the museum, or to Walt Disney World. But now, because of all the numerous medical appointments, we simply couldn't afford anything extra, which was also an adjustment for both boys. Mike and I both scheduled time to spend one-on-one with Dalton so he wouldn't feel excluded. His world had already changed when his younger brother came along, but now, with the constant worry and focus on the EoE, Dalton's world changed even more. At times we felt guilty about not finding the right balance between the two.

> *We needed to erect protective walls around us so that we could get through all the "firsts" during that first year.*

The biggest challenges, however, were found outside our home. A simple social gathering with other families became an ordeal. We were so far from a normal family that to be with friends around food was extremely difficult. I found I was becoming resentful every time someone expressed their sympathy or said they knew what Rem was going through because they couldn't eat when they had the flu or were on a strict diet or far from home. I simply smiled and nodded, while inside my heart was bleeding from the misery. I'd say the right things, but I'd be screaming to myself, *No, you really don't know what it's like to have a child who can't eat. You still attend your socials, holiday gatherings, and family get-togethers; and by the looks of you, you really don't have a clue what's it's like to not eat. You look to me as if you know how to eat pretty well.* I began looking at people differently, especially people who were overweight. I be-

The New Normal

came quite judgmental, not because I'm that kind of person but because I was hurting for my son and for what this had done to our family.

We needed to erect protective walls around us so that we could get through all the "firsts" during that first year. People mean well. I have complete understanding for all of those who tried to offer reassuring words and kind gestures, but in that first year it was almost impossible *not* to be resentful or angry. We were trying to navigate an alternate universe that was plopped inside our normal world.

People meant well, but sometimes said completely the wrong thing. One time when I went to pick Dalton up from his summer camp, one of the moms standing by me waiting for the kids to grab all of their gear, asked me which one of our boys went to the camp. I told her Dalton. She then said, "I didn't think the other one could go because he's not able to eat and that could be a problem." Even though her words hurt me—*because really, she was right*—in that moment, I realized if I allowed it to be a problem then it would be. I decided, then and there, to use the hurt to prove her and everyone else wrong. Sometimes it's the unkind things that chisel little bits and pieces of us away, but that little bit of chiseling sharpened my stone and made me stronger to face more ugliness along the way. It also fostered my

Home Plate

determination to find a way around obstacles so Remington could participate in any activity or camp that he wanted to, such as traveling to the Dominican Republic and later England and Scotland. Still, there were rough days, not just for Remington, but for all of us.

The very thing that had kept us together was our family time, our bond around the plate at the dinner table.

" *When I was little, I was confused and angry about my diagnosis. One morning, as I went into Sunday school class, my teacher at the time, Ms. Shamaine (my friend Cameren's mom) bent down to greet me. "Hello, little Remington," she said. Instead of greeting her back, I kicked her in the shin. I was wearing cowboy boots that morning and that sharp little kick caused her to almost double over in pain. My parents made me apologize, and I still feel bad about that morning, but it was a moment of frustration for a little boy who didn't understand why his world had suddenly changed so much."*

Mike and I began drifting apart from each other as well. A child with an illness puts incredible pressure on a couple. Compound that with the fact both boys

The New Normal

were young and the medical bills were enormous, our marriage began to suffer. A wonderful couple from our church invited us to attend a marriage conference with Dr. Gary Chapman, the author of *The Five Love Languages*. I was worried about leaving Remington with my parents for the weekend, but I also knew Mike and I needed to get away. It turned out to be the best decision ever.

When Dr. Chapman took a break, he offered to speak individually with couples for a brief amount of time. I jumped in that line and was later so glad I did!

It was a rather small conference and, thankfully, it didn't take much time for me to make my way to him to share our situation. It all poured out—the frustration, the meals in our bedroom, the stress. Dr. Chapman listened and then advised the way we were treating Remington was causing our family to revolve around him. We were actually making Remington the center of our existence, neglecting our older son, Dalton, as well as our marriage. Wow! He was so right. The very thing that had kept us together was our family time, our bond around the plate at the dinner table. That was our nucleus and where we caught up with one another and built our family's foundation. We lost all of that when Remington was diagnosed and food became the enemy.

Home Plate

Dr. Chapman said that, even though we meant well, we were destroying our family and were well on our way to destroying our marriage. He recommended starting to change that by gathering around the table and having dinner together again as a family. He stressed that we must teach Remington that, while his disease is unfortunate, life is not always fair. He told us to emphasize Rem has his form of nutrition now and we must have ours. He also suggested we get used to eating as a family again by adding a conversation starter where each person took a turn answering a question. That way, the focus wasn't on our food but on each other and our family conversation around the dinner table.

I couldn't wait to get home to the boys and try this out. It wasn't as easy as it sounded, but we did return to sitting at the table again as a family. We chose to avoid snack type foods and dessert treats and decided to only cook foods that would nourish our bodies. At dinner time, we would gather around the table, say grace, and begin our questions with a conversation starter. Remington understood that he wasn't to get up from the table until he had finished his shake for dinner. Sometimes, he would find himself seated at the table a bit longer than anyone else but he quickly learned that his need for nutrition was a non-negotiable. Of course, there were the occasional fits of screaming and pushing his shake box out of his reach to avoid drinking it, but

The New Normal

day by day—just as God promised—our lives became a bit more hopeful.

Our very first Thanksgiving with Remington in his foodless world, we decided to go camping. We had camped regularly since the boys were babies and we loved being able to just get away from it all. We originally spent the Thanksgiving holidays around a table with family and tons of food. However, that year Remington had just been removed from foods only a month before and we were still struggling as a family, so we thought it best to venture out. It turned out to be one of our best decisions. We focused on our family time, playing board games and card games, or simply sitting by the campfire talking and sharing memories. Remington was learning to reach for that shake when he got hungry. That Thanksgiving we were not feeling so thankful because we were still coping with our pain and Remington's losses. That Thanksgiving we didn't have a big celebratory meal either. We simply ate ham sandwiches while we played cornhole and it turned out to be one of our best holidays ever.

After that first Thanksgiving when we went camping, we planned our hospital trips to Cincinnati around Thanksgiving break so I wouldn't miss school. We stayed at my cousin's home in Columbus, which was a lot of fun because I've

Home Plate

always been close with all my family up there, especially my cousin Emma. She's only a year and a half older than me and has always been more of a sister than a cousin.

Every Thanksgiving, their family has an annual ritual: they go up to the local high school football field and kick field goals. Since we're usually up there, we get to tag along and join in. Later, when I learned to sit at the dinner table with my shakes, we began joining them at their holiday meal, too.

Tears came to my eyes just looking at the menu, knowing Rem wouldn't be able to order off a menu like that, maybe ever again.

Ohio often gets snow in November and we Florida boys loved playing in the snow. One time, Emma, Dalton and I made a snowman in her front yard, using sticks for arms. We were so proud of our creation. As we were telling our families to come look at our snowman, Emma's dog Duchess ran over, grabbed the snowman's stick arm and ran around the yard. We all began chasing after Duchess in the snow to get the snowman's arm back. Everyone was laughing and it was such a wonderful, normal, family moment."

Eventually, we went back to cooking in the kitchen. Sometimes, Remington would come up and ask to smell the food. Once I had the foods on the plate, he would actually breathe in each food item and he would say, "I remember what that tastes like." Those are the knot-forming-in-your-throat moments. Those times when, as a parent, you're trying to be strong so your child doesn't see your own weakness. Or your tears.

At times, Dalton felt guilty for being able to eat. I struggled when it came to grocery shopping. Do I buy the Cheez-It crackers for Dalton? I was afraid Remington would try to eat them too. The same thing for the cereal or the lunch meat or the cheese. How was I supposed to shop for groceries anymore? I found myself walking the aisles and seeing other families shopping together. How would we ever do that now?

Then came the challenge of dining out. Before the diagnosis, good report cards meant the boys could choose a restaurant for a celebratory meal. Dalton's favorite place to go was Red Lobster. His report card came home and it was fantastic. He was so excited to go out to his favorite restaurant. Mike and I debated but ultimately decided we should keep the tradition. We packed a lunch

Home Plate

box for Remington and set off to Red Lobster. This was the first time we had dined out since Rem's diagnosis. It was so hard. Tears came to my eyes just looking at the menu, knowing Rem wouldn't be able to order off a menu like that, maybe ever again.

I brought our conversation starter flip chart and placed it on the table. We ordered our food and began sharing about our day. Dalton was so excited, proud of his grades and of this moment about him. We ate our meals and then Dalton asked if he could have dessert. For a normal family, that's an easy answer—but for us, dessert was anything but easy. When Dalton's chocolate cake came out with whipped cream and a cherry, I saw the look on Rem's face that said plainly, *I want some.* We tried to focus on the conversation starter, but we all watched Dalton devour his dessert and silently wished for just a bite of that chocolate gooey-ness.

The very first birthday party we had for Remington in his foodless world was when he turned five. We decided to have the party at the bowling alley so the kids could keep busy and not focus so much on eating. Instead of having pizza, chips, soda, and cake we rented a snow cone machine and brought it to the bowling alley. When it came time to sing happy birthday, we gave Rem a snow cone with a candle in it.

The New Normal

I remember hearing kids ask where the cake was and seeing some parents huddled together enquiring about the food. For us, this was our new normal. For them, this was a moment they shared in Remington's new world. That first public birthday celebration hit Mike and I hard. We both choked up when kids sang "Happy Birthday" to Rem. It was a tough, heart-wrenching moment for us. Some of the parents who hadn't known about Remington's disease until that moment were sympathetic and emotional.

 I remember my mom and dad taking turns to come to my school for class parties and going with me when my friends had birthday parties. The first class party was the hardest and most painful. During all the excitement and fuss over a cupcake, candy, and punch, my mom took my hand and led me to the bookshelf so that I could read with her. What kid wants to read a book instead of eating a cupcake or candy? My mom could have taken me home instead of making me sit there, but my parents were tough on me because they knew I needed to learn how to navigate through the many food situations that I would have to face.

My mom also sent in non-food treats to school, like pencils, baseball cards, erasers, sticker packs,

Home Plate

Matchbox cars, and little bouncy balls so the teacher could hand those out as treats/rewards. Mom also made up little goodie bags for me when she knew there was a birthday party. That way, I could be handed that one instead of the one filled with candy and I wouldn't feel excluded.

> It gave him a small measure of control over something other kids took for granted and allowed others a glimpse into his world.

Then there was Halloween, Thanksgiving, and Christmas. For Halloween, my parents decided to pay me a quarter for each piece of candy I got. Then we'd count it and they would take me to the store so I could buy something. Dalton loved this plan because I would give him all of my candy after we counted it.

At a Christmas party at school, my dad took time off of work to join me. The class was decorating cookies. I'd decorate mine and my dad immediately ate it. As much as possible, my parents tried to keep my life normal. I'm not saying it wasn't hard to not eat those cookies, but my parents did

The New Normal

their best to ease that pain and keep me from feeling 'different'."

We decided to let Remington decide what we'd have for his birthday celebrations. If he didn't want food then we wouldn't have food. It gave him a small measure of control over something other kids took for granted and allowed others a glimpse into his world.

As each birthday passed, we discovered we'd become more active and creative in deciding where we held his parties. One birthday was spent on a pirate cruise, one playing laser tag, and yet another at an airsoft field. Even though Rem's birthday is in January and it might be a bit cold, each birthday's dessert was a snow cone.

We learned to celebrate without food. We learned to focus on what was important, not on a cake or ice cream. We no longer gathered around the table for a formal celebratory meal. We left food out on the table and when the guests were hungry they'd grab a bite while Rem drank his shake. Then off they'd go again, playing manhunt in the woods or swimming in the pool. It got easier, but still we hurt for our child, who was left out of a rite of passage.

When Rem was invited to birthday parties, he would go to the ones that involved some type of activity or outing like tubing, airsoft, or going to the movies, and he'd bring his lunch box filled with shakes. As time went on, he began to be comfortable around food and comfortable with his disease.

We might not have been sitting down to eat cake or passing the peas to Rem, but our plates were full. Full of first time experiences like these that really caused us to hurt in our hearts and made lumps form in our throats from holding back the tears. Mike and I would watch Rem, a hundred unspoken questions between us.

What did the future hold? What would life be like for Rem? What will it be like when he starts dating? What will others think?

Questions aside, we were full of faith; secure in the knowledge that God doesn't give us any more than we can handle and only enough to challenge us so we become stronger. When our strength wavered, we reached out to God to shore us up.

Most of all, though, our family was full of love and a hope that continues to keep us fighting for life and a cure. That hope keeps us going, ready for the days to come and whatever challenges they might hold.

The New Normal

Home Plate

Part Two

As told by Remington Walls with comments from his parents Stephanie and Mike.

Home Plate

Chapter 5:

Baseball and Art

Eosinophilic Esophagitis.

The diagnosis made me angry. I was four years old and forbidden to eat any and all foods because my esophagus was failing. I didn't quite comprehend what that meant at that age, but I knew that something about me was going to be different—that *I* was different from everyone else. I had endured all of these scary tests and doctor visits, and now . . .

More.

The more meant drinking a formula every day. Bitter and tart and constant. I could barely hold it down and hated every sip for the longest time. I had no other choices—there was no "eat this and you can have some cake" or "try a bite and you can have the chicken nuggets instead". It was eat this or, for all intents and purposes, you will die.

Home Plate

Maybe that's part of why I was so angry. My choices were gone.

> One day when Remington was eight years old, I had gotten angry with him for something. I can't remember about what, but I'll never forget what happened afterward. Rem came up with his suitcase all packed, clutching his Mickey Mouse under his arm. He told me that he was leaving. When I asked him why, he said it was because I didn't appreciate him and that he was going to find a new family that would. Evidently, his little love tank was on empty. As hard as it was for me, I helped him open the front and screen doors. I bent down and gave him a hug and kiss and told him I loved him. As he began walking down the front walkway and away from our home, I asked him if he packed any shakes to take with him. He turned around and said no. I said, "Well hold up, let me get you a case." I grabbed a case and walked it out to him. There he was with his suitcase in one hand and Mickey in the other. He looked at me, sighed deeply, and then

Maybe that's part of why I was so angry. My choices were gone.

Baseball and Art

> *said, "Well, I guess I'll give you another chance to appreciate me 'cuz I don't know how I'm supposed to carry all of this stuff." I went with him to his room and helped him unpack his suitcase."*

My parents took me to counseling and enrolled me in art class so I could express my feelings. I didn't want to go to art and I remember kicking and screaming, trying to get out of the classes. My mom insisted, though, saying art classes would help me express all the emotions I kept bottled up inside me. So, for two days a week I sat in a classroom and drew.

My first pictures were dark and scary, full of black and gray. My mom never acted like the pictures were anything different and hung them on the fridge, regardless. Dark circles, trees, buildings . . . for weeks, that was all I created.

One day, I got in the car, handed my drawing to my mother, and she began to cry. I didn't understand why she was upset so I asked her why she was crying. She looked down at the picture, and sobbed, "Because you added yellow."

At the time I had no idea what she meant. When I got older, I realized that splash of yellow indicated a shift in my attitude. For the first time in a long time, my parents saw I was beginning to emotionally deal with my disease, and my anger was beginning to ease. I went to art classes for two years and drew lions, tigers, and monkeys. One tiger picture I drew, I gave to my doctor, Dr. P at Cincinnati Children's Hospital. It was my way of thanking him for helping me feel better. He hung it near the front door of the clinic office.

One day, I got in the car, handed my drawing to my mother, and she began to cry.

" *I believe those art lessons helped Remington share his emotions and learn to understand what he was feeling at the time. When he first started lessons, his pictures were dark. He didn't use any color at all. Each time I would pick him up, I was hopeful it would be the day he finally added a touch of color. Then one day, there was a tiny bit of yellow in one of his pictures. Tears came to my eyes as I thought finally, a turning point. Our boy was returning to us. Then came the family picture with all of us smiling. I knew then that we were on the right path, especially since Remington had drawn himself with a smile."*

Baseball and Art

What really changed my life was baseball. I loved baseball! I'd be ready to go before anyone else in the house, sitting on the steps with my cap on my head and my glove on my hand. When I wasn't on the field playing, I played in the front yard with my brother, my dad, or even by myself. I had a little plastic bat and ball and four tiny little bases, but it was enough. I loved everything about baseball—running, hitting, catching, and throwing. Every spare second, I had, I played baseball.

My parents were my biggest cheerleaders. They told me baseball seemed to be my natural God-given ability and supported me, no matter how far the drive or how long the practice. They told Dalton and I that we could be anything we wanted to be and that there were no limitations to what either one of us could do.

Like any kid, I didn't always remember those words of encouragement or the joy I found in baseball. I remember one time when I was feeling really down about myself. I was having a pity party because we were back at Cincinnati Children's Hospital for yet another endoscopy to see if I had passed or failed a food trial.

My mom made me sit beside her in the lobby. After a few minutes of silence, she asked me what I noticed about the people that I saw.

Home Plate

"I see a girl in a wheelchair. She doesn't have any legs."

"Okay," Mom said. "What else do you see?"

I looked around the lobby. "I see a boy hooked up to a machine, walking down the hall and pushing his machine with him." For a few minutes, I pointed out the different people walking by, people with all kinds of injuries and disabilities.

> "Right now, you have a choice," she placed her hands on my shoulders. "You can let your disease control your life or you can choose to live your life, regardless of your disease."

Finally, my mother asked me, "What do people see when they see you?"

"They don't see anything wrong with me," I said. It was true—from the outside, I looked like any other kid. I didn't have a missing limb or a machine to help me live. I dressed, walked, talked, and looked like everyone else. The only time I was "different" was when I had to drink formula for a meal instead of eating cereal or a cheeseburger.

Baseball and Art

"You're right, Remington," she nodded. Then she turned to me, making sure I was looking into her eyes before she went on. "There is nothing wrong with you. The only thing you can't do is eat the same food we do, but you've been blessed with another source of nutrition. You're complaining about having another endoscopy but the children you've seen today can't play baseball like you can."

I thought of that girl in the wheelchair and the boy dragging the machine behind him. Other kids were lying in hospital beds or hooked up to oxygen tanks.

"Right now, you have a choice," she placed her hands on my shoulders. "You can let your disease control your life or you can choose to live your life, regardless of your disease."

I could choose to live my life. In all the years since, that moment has stuck with me. I have chosen to live life, even when I've had endoscopy number fifty-seven or opened up my thousandth box of formula. In those moments, I remind myself that I'm really blessed and to be grateful for the life I have.

I loved baseball because my Dad introduced me to it, but I think another one of the reasons why I loved baseball so much is that on the field I'm not Remington with

Home Plate

EoE—I'm not that kid that drinks some weird formula thing. I'm just me.

When I was eight years old, I met one of my closest friends, Matt, on the field. So many of the boys I played with at a young age stayed friends with me all through school, both on and off the field. There's Edgar, whom I met playing on my high school team, and then Cameren, whose father was one of my coaches. Cameren's mom, Shamaine, nicknamed me "Twinkle Toes" because I was the fastest runner on the team. Cameren and I played on a competitive team for three years and then on the high school All-Star team in our senior year.

As soon as I came off the field, however, I was back to being the "different" kid. We'd come in for a snack after practice or a game and all the other kids sat around munching on a granola bar and guzzling a Gatorade. Most of the time the parents didn't know I couldn't eat so I'd just say, "no thank you" or "I'm good". Sometimes I took the snack they gave me just to avoid any question why I didn't want one or to forestall any urgings to take the stuff anyway. I'd stuff the snack in my pocket and give it to my dad or brother later. When I got older, it was easier because I was secure in myself and in what my disease meant, but it was hard as a seven or eight-year-old to feel excluded and have everyone won-

Baseball and Art

der why I didn't want any snacks. My parents bought me baseball cards as a postgame treat, but it wasn't the same.

When Remington began playing ball, he was so enthusiastic that he raced out of the dugout, his glove already on. He wanted to be the first out there. At times, he would sing and swing his glove around when he was on base. It was a sign he was finally happy again. Happy because his body didn't hurt anymore. Happy because he was doing something he loved. Whenever he was on the field, he seemed to be energized and excited. As time passed, he became more skilled and focused. Every day, he spent hours working on fielding grounders and hitting. If he wasn't at the high school practicing then he'd be in our yard working with Mike. He seemed to live and breathe baseball.

When Remington played competitive baseball, we found it easier not to say anything about his disease. He attended every practice and participated just like everyone else. However, sometimes running in the heat became too much for him because of his shake intake or he'd throw up after running sprints. On double-header days, Rem often drank sugar water to gain some needed ener-

gy. I remember watching the boys run and would grow concerned for Rem, who had said he didn't want us to say anything so we kept quiet. I'll never forget the day the coach told Rem he'd never play baseball in high school. I guarantee you, we did not keep out mouths shut then. Was it because Rem was different and not like everyone else? Did this coach view Rem in a different light? Looking back, we are grateful for his harshness because he gave us a glimpse into what the real world was like and how they view people who are different. It taught us what discrimination looked and sounded like. Rem later played for a competitive team that had a feeling of family togetherness. He played three years for this team and the coach saw Rem as an inspiration, not as "different". That made a difference for Rem and for the team as a whole."

At team parties, I'd stay in the pool or go talk to my dad until everyone got their food, and then I would go sit back down with my friends. It was awkward because only my closest friends on the team knew why I wasn't eating. I didn't want to explain over and over again and I didn't want to be "different". By the time I was thirteen and playing on the travel team, almost everyone on the team was someone I played with growing up so

Baseball and Art

they already knew about my EoE and were comfortable with it.

Not everyone understood my disease, and not everyone treated me like the rest of the team. At one weekend tournament, the coach made the whole team run sprints. It was ninety degrees. I had just finished one of my shakes—which has a milk-like thickness. It's my only nutrition for the day, so it's not like I can run and grab a Powerbar or a Gatorade to replace it. Imagine running sprints in the heat of the sun after drinking two glasses of milk. That's what it was like for me that day.

The most invaluable lesson I have gained from baseball is to work hard. To power through any situation.

I threw up and my energy level was almost zero, which happens often with EoE. I don't get the energy boost other people do from eating regular food. Sometimes during doubleheaders, I drank sugar water to boost my energy level. Most of the time, I simply pushed myself harder to fight through the fatigue.

That day, however, after the game we had just played, the heat, the sprints, along with the lack of nutrition in my body after I got sick—it was just too much. The coach saw me as lazy, and when I tried to explain, he didn't want to hear it. He cut me from the team.

I credit that coach with teaching me a harsh lesson about what discrimination can be like. I was different and he didn't want to understand. Later, he learned more about EoE, realized why I had been struggling so much, and invited me back to the team. I stayed for a few more tournaments, but moved to another team—one that embraced me.

The most invaluable lesson I have gained from baseball is to work hard. To power through any situation. I believe that hard work beats talent on any given day. Now, don't get me wrong—there's always going to be someone more talented than you, but talent can only take you so far. I'm driven to play baseball and do something every day to work toward that goal.

Baseball was something that I could control, unlike the disease that tried to control me. I control my ability to play. I control how much I give in practice or on game day. I control my attitude and my teamwork. And in return, baseball gives me a joy that makes up for every one of those trips to the hospital.

Chapter 6:

School Days

> *There were a lot of questions. I was different, and when you're young, being different is an open invitation for ridicule.*

It's the little things that helped me feel a little less excluded when I was young: My uncle Ron gave me an ice machine so I could have a snow-cone, leading my parents to bring an ice machine to my fifth birthday. Everyone at the party, including me, had sno-cones instead of cake. Dressing up as a pilgrim for the Thanksgiving celebration at my elementary school. Spending the night at my friend Peyton's house. I wanted so desperately to look and feel "normal" but every time I had to get out a shake and drink it, I knew I was anything but.

When I was young, it was hard for my parents to let me go to other kids' homes by myself because they were afraid I might eat something. Plus, it took a lot

Home Plate

of planning just to go—there were the shakes to pack, the schedule to review, and the plan to come get me if I felt tired or out of place. My lunchbox, which held my shakes, went with me everywhere. To school, the store, my friends' houses. It would have been easier if I stayed at home. My mom worried the most about what would happen when I wasn't under their watchful eye, but my dad convinced her that allowing me to go out in the world alone would be good for me.

In fourth grade, I switched from private school to public school, leaving behind all the kids I'd known since Pre-K. Private school was like a bubble—every part of the day was managed: your classes, your behavior, and even what you wore. I soon realized public school was a whole new world. Kids said and wore what they wanted. They had no filter. Again, my mom scheduled a day to come into talk to the class about me and explained why I could only drink shakes. There were a lot of questions. I was different, and when you're young, being different is an open invitation for ridicule. For the most part, the kids I went to school with were more curious than mean.

The first time I pulled out my shake to drink it in class, the kids around me were surprised and curious. They kept asking me, "What does it taste like?" The flavor is too hard to explain so I'd just let them try

School Days

it. One sip, and they were rinsing out their mouths. I couldn't blame them. That bitter, weird taste is hard to ignore.

Surprisingly, it was adults I encountered who could be less than understanding. One day in fourth grade, we had a substitute teacher. My regular teacher (who was and still is my favorite teacher), was out for the day. School started around 9 a.m., so I'd have my first shake around 10:30. I reached down and took my shake out of my lunchbox like I had done every day. Business as usual, and all the kids in class had gotten so used to it they didn't even notice anymore. I started shaking it, and just as I put in the straw to take my first sip, the sub walked over and said, "You're not allowed to drink that right now; it's not lunchtime." She took it out of my hand and put it on top of a high bookshelf, too high for a four-foot tall fourth grader to reach. I tried explaining to her that I needed to drink it, that I couldn't wait until lunchtime. My classmate Briana, spoke up too and tried to explain, but the sub wouldn't listen.

> *"You were chosen for a reason," he said. "I don't know what that reason is, but I do know you're going to have to be tougher than the circumstances life throws at you."*

Home Plate

I started to panic. I knew I had to drink the shakes on a regular schedule so that my body could have time to process each one before the next one was due. This teacher ignored us and I wasn't sure I could wait two more hours to eat. Briana went across the hall and got another teacher, one who knew about my disease and explained the situation to the sub but it was too late. I was beyond humiliated. I went to the bathroom, locked the door, and just sat on the floor and cried.

I was still crying when I got home, questioning why I was chosen to live with this, to be different. My dad sat down beside me. "You were chosen for a reason," he said. "I don't know what that reason is, but I do know you're going to have to be tougher than the circumstances life throws at you. One bad chapter doesn't define the book."

The next morning, I stalled getting ready for school. What if that sub was there again? What if people asked me about what happened? I didn't want to go to school for the rest of the week, or the week after, or ever again. I was still so embarrassed to have been the center of attention like that, to be in that panicked moment of not knowing what to do. My mom came in my room and sat on the edge of my bed. "If you don't go to school, Rem, you'll hide," she said. "And then

School Days

you'll be hiding for the rest of your life, running from every hard time life throws at you."

I tried to argue but she made me go to school. That day, my regular teacher was back. She felt terrible because she'd forgotten to leave a note about me for the sub. She gave me a huge hug and apologized over and over. The school day went on and life got back to normal, but I've never forgotten that day.

In middle school, my mom worked at the school and kept my shakes in the fridge in her classroom. Between classes, I would grab one and then go to class. I could have gone to the nurse's office every time, but my parents taught me I needed to stay in class, plus the teachers didn't mind me drinking in class because staying meant I didn't miss any of the material. The only awkward time in school was lunch. My friends would get into the line to get their lunches and I'd sit at the table by myself until they got back. Everyone at school knew I couldn't eat but it still felt weird just sitting there by myself, drinking my box of formula.

As the school years went on, things got easier and more routine. Most of the kids from middle school went to my high school, which made the transition for me much easier since they already knew about my

Home Plate

EoE. Luckily, one of our family friends worked at the school and let me keep my shakes in her room. No teenager wants to walk around with a lunchbox full of juice boxes, so I was glad I could stop by Ms. Amy's room throughout the day.

In freshman year, I met my best friend, Edgar Vasquez. We both loved baseball, liked the same music—everything. To this day, we still do everything together. We were on homecoming court together, prom court together, and played on the county Allstar team together. Most of my friends played sports, too—Dave played basketball, Matt played football, and Ethan played hockey. We went to each other's games and were the loudest ones in the crowd cheering each other on. Dakota was my workout partner. We've always been the first ones in and the last ones out. Our motto was that no one would outwork us. We pushed each other to always be better and to continue to get better. We were up while everyone was sleeping and were practicing while everyone else was hanging around. Dakota always helped me stay focused, even when things fell apart for a while.

> *I've learned to laugh at myself, and with others, and that has made some truly difficult times so much more bearable.*

These guys are my brothers and I love them to death. Just as Briana did that day in fourth grade, my friends have stepped in whenever anyone said anything. My parents helped make it easy by investing their time early on to educate others and to not allow me to be seen as a sick kid who needed special treatment because of my EoE. Maybe it was because of that, or because I was cool with what my life has been, but I was never bullied or made fun of in school. My friends are now so comfortable with the shakes that they tease me, asking me dopy questions like, *because you only drink liquid, does that mean you only pee?* I'd answer and say nope. My liquid is food and so I do everything you all do.

One time, when we were making a film segment for a Neocate informational video on my EoE (which was filmed at my school's baseball field), my friend Spencer grabbed one of my shakes and pretended to be me drinking from it. He got my mannerisms down and everything, even the way that I chomp down on my straw and hang it off the side of my mouth. All of us—Edgar, Dakota, me—burst out laughing. I looked around at this group of guys and thought of how blessed I have been, not just with my family, but with them, too. I've learned to laugh at myself, and with others, and that has made some truly difficult times so much more bearable.

Chapter 7:

Almost Quitting

"You have a torn labrum," the doctor said, and for the first time since my EoE diagnosis, I was scared, depressed, and worried my life would never be the same again.

I was a freshman in high school, and only a few weeks into baseball season and my first Junior Varsity team. About halfway through the season, my shoulder started to hurt. I chalked it up to fatigue and took some time off from throwing, filling in as the designated hitter for a while. One week of rest, no change. Two weeks, no change. Three weeks, no change. The pain was still there.

I lay on the MRI table, a thousand "what ifs" running through my head. Baseball was a major part of my life. It was the one place in the world where I felt strong, capable, and just like any other kid. Then the doctor pointed out the torn labrum and I heard phrases like physical therapy and possible surgery.

Home Plate

I tried six weeks of PT and nothing changed. The doctor recommended another six weeks, but there was still no change. I could see the season ticking by, with me mostly in the dugout instead of out on the field.

I prayed about my shoulder and had a lot of conversations with God about what I was going through. At one point, a peace about the whole thing came over me. At my next appointment, I told the doctor, "Let's do the surgery. I know I'm going to come out of this okay."

He stared at me, then said, "There's a very good chance you won't be able to throw again."

I know it's all part of His plan. I may not understand it; I don't have to understand it. I just have to trust it.

I thought of all those hospital visits I had undergone. The tests. The years of shakes and food trials and frustration. God pulled me through all of that, so I knew He would pull me through this, too. "No," I said to the doctor, "you've got the wrong guy. Other people might not be able to throw again, but that's not me."

I have always taken comfort in Jeremiah 29:11: "For I know the plans I have for you, declares the Lord, plans to prosper you and not to harm you, plans to give you

Almost Quitting

hope and a future." That's the same verse I've recited to myself every day of my life, and because of that I don't stress over anything—I know it's all part of His plan. I may not understand it; I don't have to understand it. I just have to *trust* it.

On surgery day, I knew I had God on my side. They wheeled me back and strapped me down to the table. The doctor walked in and asked, "You ready?"

The anesthesia was starting to work, but I gave him a thumbs-up. "Doc G, I got the easy part." Then it was lights out.

I woke up in the recovery room with my arm in a sling, extended out like I was about to shake hands. My dad told me the doctor had to put anchors and sutures in my arm, but everything had gone as well as it could. I was confident I would come through this like I had everything else.

Then we got home and the pain medications wore off. All of a sudden, it felt like a hot knife was driving deeper and deeper into my shoulder. My mom gave me another dose and I started to feel better. Just as I was about to doze off in the recliner (I couldn't sleep in a bed because of the way my arm was extended and for fear that

Home Plate

I would roll over and tear my repair), I felt the worst pain in my stomach.

That wasn't good. I knew that from all the times I was in Cincinnati Children's Hospital. I began vomiting repeatedly and freaked out. I thought it was something to do with my EoE, but it turned out I was allergic to the pain medication. Imagine dealing with the pain of surgery and then vomiting all over the place. I was miserable. That was basically life saying "Good luck, Rem. You're on your own and without any pain meds. Have fun with that." I went through an eight-month rehab process with no pain medication, and I'm not going to lie—it was horrible, and there were times when I wanted to break because of the pain. Later, my physical therapist recommended a specially made prescription pain cream which helped a lot.

All I'd wanted to do in high school was play baseball and my first season was over before it even started.

Before the surgery, my dad warned me the repair was the easy part—rehab would be the hard part. He was right. I spent four weeks in a sling so I wouldn't tear the anchors out of place, then started PT. My physical therapist, Kim, stretched my arms over my head, across my chest, and the pain was so incredibly bad. I spent

Almost Quitting

the first couple months just trying to get my range of motion back. I sometimes got frustrated, knowing I was missing my freshman year of baseball. I was determined to be at 100% for my sophomore season. I saw Kim three days a week and she told me I'd improve faster if I did my exercises every day. "The more you do it, the quicker you'll bounce back."

So, every morning I'd wake up at 4:30 to stretch and strengthen before going to school. then I still went to baseball practice and watched, but all I wanted to do was be out there. When I got home in the evenings, I'd immediately head to our home gym to do my exercises before going to bed. Because it was tough going in those early weeks and months, my dad would sit in my room and push me when I worked on my physical therapy. Sometimes helping me lift my arm into the proper position.

I remember I couldn't even slide a small soup can across the counter at first. Then, as I kept going, I could lift small weights: first out to the side, and then above my head. I'd see my friends on the field and feel the frustration and pain of the slow road back, then I'd get depressed and weaken. All I'd wanted to do in high school was play baseball and my first season was over before it even started.

Home Plate

"When it was time for high school, Remington was thrilled. He couldn't wait to play high school ball. Unfortunately, that dream was short lived during his freshman year. His shoulder surgery was another setback but it proved to be a pivotal turning point in his life. At the age of fourteen, Remington discovered who he really was and how powerful his mind could be. When he was four, his father and I were the ones pushing him onward. Now it was time for him to push himself. His fighting spirit kicked in and he fought through the pain of recovery—without any pain medication. I'd hear his alarm go off at 4:30 in the morning and then hear him moaning and fighting to do his stretches. As a mother, it's tough to witness your child struggle. I wanted to help him, but I knew he had to do this on his own. Sometimes, I found myself standing by his door and praying that his pain would lessen."

> I changed my mindset and decided winning was a conscious choice. I needed to make that choice every single day, during every single repetition.

Almost Quitting

I started listening to motivational videos. I was at the lowest point in my life but listening to them and hearing the passion in their voices lit a fire in me to push myself beyond my breaking point. Eric Thomas was one of my favorites. He said things like, "Don't cry to quit, cry to keep going." Those were the words that helped me find the fire inside myself to make it through. I would do my exercises, tearing and rebuilding that scar tissue, all the while crying from the deep, agonizing pain, and looking for any excuse to quit, then Thomas or someone else would say something that would get me back on track.

"Pain is temporary," Eric Thomas said, and I took that to heart because, no matter how bad it got, I knew one day the pain would be gone—and on the other side of pain, success was waiting. I changed my mindset and decided winning was a conscious choice. I needed to make that choice every single day, during every single repetition.

When it was time for me to begin throwing, my parents hired Larry Mayol, a former trainer for the New York Mets. He wasn't just my trainer—he became a man I trusted. He has a deep faith and a wealth of stories that offered me encouragement and kept me pushing forward. I respect him greatly to this day.

Home Plate

The road back to throwing would be just as difficult as regaining my range of motion. I had lost all the muscle on my upper body. Larry showed me a picture of my back—out of shape, no longer defined, and weakened. Then he showed me a picture of another kid's back who had the same surgery. This kid was muscular, shredded and strong. "This is what your back will look like in four weeks if you do the work," Larry said, lighting a fire inside of me.

I worked with Larry for months getting my strength back and learning to throw again. I wouldn't be where I am today without Larry and his wealth of knowledge. I still go to him to this day, and our bond is unbreakable. He's been a blessing to me and my family.

I spent a lot of time at home during those eight months, afraid to get hurt or damage my arm. I felt disconnected from my friends and was glad when sophomore year started.

My coach met with me and two other guys to inform us he was going to give us a shot on the varsity team. I was pumped but also worried—I hadn't played in a game in almost a year. Our first game rolled around and we were playing one of the best teams in the county. Finally, my first at-bat and my anxiety got the better of me. I was so worried about proving to the coach that I

Almost Quitting

belonged there that I put too much pressure on myself to perform . . .

And I struck out in three pitches. That moment tore my confidence apart and I faltered every time I was at the plate. I finished the fall hitting about .210. After the last preseason game, the coach pulled me aside and told me I was going to be on JV instead. I was crushed because I knew I could've done better. That spring I doubled down, working harder every game and started hitting over .300. I received the JV Offensive Player Award, but what I really wanted was that varsity slot.

It didn't happen. I was benched for almost the entire season my junior year because I wasn't good enough. I had one at-bat and spent maybe four innings in the field. It got to the point where I didn't even want to go on game days because I felt useless just sitting there on the bench. My parents told me that riding the bench teaches humility, but that was really tough on me. And as much as I didn't want to be there, I did want to be there for my teammates. These guys were my brothers and I wanted to support them. Every game I watched, every pitch and hit I saw, added wood to the fire, as Michael Jordan would say. I was determined to improve, get a spot on that varsity team, and play.

Home Plate

" *I was so excited for Remington's senior year to be here. In September, Remington and I had been invited to speak at a Neocate conference in Minnesota to share his story about growing up on their product. He shared the ups and downs of living his life with formula only and some of the obstacles that he's had to overcome because of it. Rem thoroughly enjoyed speaking to an audience and he was a natural.*

When we returned, I couldn't wait for baseball to start.

> The EoE doesn't define who I am. It has only made me stronger. And when I falter, I'm reminded once again of Jeremiah 29:11.

The home games were especially memorable because Mike was the official griller. Our extended family would show up to watch the game. We'd sit over by the third base side and cheer the boys on. On Remington's senior night, all of our family was there in support and even some of the folks from Neocate came, as well. This was a sign that Rem's final season would be over soon. Another chapter in our book closed and new ones beginning. As I watched Remington, I couldn't help but think of

Almost Quitting

how far we had come. How dark those first years were and how much brighter things are now."

Senior season, I made a decision to work harder. I woke up at four o'clock every morning and would be in my garage a half hour later to work out before school. After school, I'd stay and hit in the cage and take groundballs. I have trouble gaining weight because my only "food" is the formula I drink, so I decided my best option was to be one of the strongest kids on the team. I doubted anyone else was doing what I was doing because few high schoolers were going to be up that early or staying that late after practice to work more.

I found that hard work, works. I finished my senior year hitting right around .300. After not playing during my junior season, I was chosen for the county Allstar team and received recognition at the Allstar banquet as well as the Most Improved Player award from my high school team. In school, my life was going great, too. I was chosen for prom court and nominated as a finalist for Outstanding Senior by my peers.

I think all these great things happened because I refused to quit. My belief was bigger than my circumstance. I didn't allow my disease to get in the way of my goals. The EoE doesn't define who I am. It has only made me stronger. And when I falter, I'm reminded once again of Jeremiah 29:11.

I owe much to the people who helped me along the way: Dr. G, Kim, Larry, and great coaches like Coach Baisley and Coach May who taught me to become a better player. Every day, they were out there coaching me and the other guys. Giving instruction on our mistakes and our attitudes. I'm also thankful to Coach Gwinn and Coach Wilcox for their commitment. But in the end, the only one with the power to come back from that surgery and be the player I wanted to be was me. I could have taken it easy or used the EoE as an excuse not to give it my all, but I didn't want to live a half-life—no way could I just give half to the things I did and expect to live fully. So, I became determined to give my all to everything I did and then use what I had been blessed with to give back to others.

Chapter 8:

Accepting Help

It's not easy to accept help, but sometimes it's necessary. I had to learn that lesson after my shoulder surgery, when doing simple things was almost impossible. And I also had to learn that when our insurance stopped covering the only sustenance I had— that elemental formula.

This was a true lesson in humility for all of us. It was also a reminder that God had it all under control.

That year, our insurance plan listed my formula as a "supplement", like a vitamin, and therefore would no longer cover the cost, which runs about $2,000 per *month*.

We made appeals arguing that this wasn't a supplement, it was a necessity. Remove the formula from my diet and all I have left to sustain me is water. A supplement is something that is added to a diet already in existence. My entire diet is elemental formula. My parents aren't

Home Plate

rich and had already struggled financially with all the medical bills. All of a sudden, they needed to come up with another two thousand a month.

A friend of our family's, Janeen, reached out and asked if we'd let her set up a Go Fund Me page. At first, my parents told her no. Janeen came back and bluntly said, "You need to swallow your pride and let us help you."

My parents realized they weren't going to be able to keep up with this massive, scary expense so they finally agreed. We were amazed by how much my friends, my school, my church, and people in the community helped us. Even my principal tweeted about it and my story later ended up on the front page of our school district's website. Our community, my school, peers, teachers, and strangers from all over rallied behind our family to donate and write encouraging messages. Even the little league park where I grew up playing ball helped by holding a fundraiser. This was a true lesson in humility for all of us. It was also a reminder that God had it all under control. Donations started to come in and my parents were so grateful.

Then the media caught wind of our situation. One day, I came home from baseball practice and found my parents sitting on the front porch. My mom said that the phone had been ringing non-stop and she wasn't an-

Accepting Help

swering it anymore. News stations had been calling all day, wanting to talk about the Go Fund Me campaign on the School District's website. Just as I sat down to talk to my dad about how practice went that day, a news van passed our house. They parked and came up to us, asking if they could talk to us. We were speechless. We weren't prepared for, and never expected, that kind of publicity.

However, that story was the turning point for me and for so many others. The formula was covered again, which was a blessing. My family and I then realized we needed to enact legislation to protect and help others like me.

We decided to partner with the American Partnership for Eosinophilic Disorders to pursue legislation. APFED had been a huge help to my family every step of my life's journey. To show our gratitude, we fundraised for them for years by hosting the Remington Walls Golf Tournament to Benefit APFED. It took a lot of time to plan and my entire family, including my Papa, Uncle Jeff, and Aunt Cissy helped us with this tournament each year. My parents wanted to create something positive out of all that had happened to our family.

Home Plate

My dad, brother, and I played in each tournament. After everyone was done golfing, they'd return to the country club for a banquet where my parents would show the video "Let Them be Little" that my mom created for APFED to help educate people about this disease. The golfers saw how their donations were being used to make a difference.

The American Partnership for Eosinophilic Disorders (APFED) has been a constant in our lives and a saving grace for our family. This organization helped us navigate through the most challenging times in our life. We found a purpose in helping others and APFED introduced us to some amazing people who were walking the same path. We were able to make connections and not feel so lost or alone during a really dark period in our lives. Some of those people who helped us were Beth, Julie, and Wendy who were key principals within the APFED organization.

Since that very first golf tournament fundraiser, we have been actively involved in APFED. In our early years, we attended the annual conferences and later helped to organize a grand rounds for doctors regarding EoE. When we realized we needed to facilitate change, APFED helped connect us to people involved in legislative efforts in

Accepting Help

other states. Their wisdom and insight has helped guide us in our pursuit to pass legislation here in Florida.

Planning these fundraising events helped our family immensely. It was the "positive" in a negative situation. We believed that when you do something kind for someone else, it makes you feel better, too, and that was true in this case.

The fundraisers were more than a way of giving back. They were also part of our educating others on this bizarre disease. We showed informational videos, answered questions, and wrote articles. Telling others about Remington, and other children like him, was our way of healing our own hurts. We were hoping to spread the word. That was our small way of making a difference.

Throughout our journey, even though we no longer hold the golf tournament fundraisers, we have remained in contact with APFED. At times, they will reach out asking for help or asking for us to make a connection to another family and we gladly connect."

Our family held this tournament for about eight years with other side fundraisers along the way. One year

Home Plate

we had "Pine View Idol"—after *American Idol* —as a fundraiser at my mom's school, which two teachers that my mom worked with, Ms. Fink and Ms. Neri, coordinated. Another year, we hosted a fundraiser kickball game between Pine View Middle, my mom's school, and my elementary school, Pine View Elementary, which teachers from both schools helped to coordinate.

> *When I realized that money was being placed above the cost of someone's life, I resolved to do something about it.*

However, when our family was hit with that massive bill for my formula, we knew we had to help change things for other families. After our story ran in newspapers and magazines, many people reached out to tell us about their experiences and hardships. So many people had lost their homes or were forced into bankruptcy—just to feed their child. Some families had no option but to have a feeding tube inserted into their otherwise healthy child because that was the only way their insurance company would cover the formula. They refused coverage if the child was actually able to drink it, forcing parents to have the child undergo an invasive procedure and receive the formula through a hole in his or her stomach. Why would you put a tube into a perfectly healthy child who can drink the formula? It seemed so unfair and it made me furious that families were forced to make decisions like that. To the insurance company, it was business as usual. After all, their decisions came down to dollars and cents—their bottom line. When I realized that money was being placed above the cost of someone's life, I resolved to do something about it.

My mom and I began meeting with state legislators about the need for legislation that would mandate formula coverage for people like me who need it for survival. We were lucky to have two senators on board to help us. A lot of time was spent on writing the language of the bill with a bill drafter. Eventually, the bill was dropped and a push for an amendment was made to an existing bill. The amendment had support on the Senate side but it ultimately failed because we weren't able to find a representative on the House side to support it. The discussion always came around to the cost. What's it going to cost the state? What's the cost to insure all these people who need it? Money once again won out.

 In June 2018, Remington and I were invited to join APFED, along with other non-profits, to advocate for formula coverage on Capitol Hill in Washington, D.C. Remington and I agreed to be actively involved in this because our hope is to

Home Plate

trump it at the state level if we can pass legislation on a federal level. We have struggled with the state of Florida to change the law and hope this might set a precedent for states that have no legislation. The bill is called the Medical Nutrition Equity Act and it calls for insurance plans to cover medical foods for children and adults. So far, there are many supporters of this bill on both the Democrat and Republican sides but we're in need of many more.

A few days before heading to D.C., Remington was asked by APFED if he would speak during a Congressional briefing session. He agreed to speak because he feels he has been walking this path for a reason, that he's been chosen. A few times, he said he was nervous because this was so important and he didn't want to mess it up. He had five minutes for his speech and had to keep it short—informative but powerful enough to make an impact, all in a few minutes.

Before we spoke with the congressmen, we met with APFED for a briefing. It was great being able to reconnect with Mary Jo Stroebel, director of APFED, and Beth Allen, one of the founders and former president of APFED. We also had many families approach us, telling us how inspirational

Accepting Help

our journey had been for them and thanking us for sharing our story with Neocate for the informational video last year. Moms shared that they watched Rem's video segment and then had their own children watch so they could see a positive outcome to their own situation. Other people came up to Remington to shake his hand and give him hugs for his honesty and encouragement. Doctors came up to shake his hand and tell him that his story was inspiring and how powerful it was to see a young man living successfully with this disease.

During this morning briefing session, we were handed our itinerary for the day and the appointments that were scheduled for us. That was a huge help. In our state meetings, I spent weeks calling and emailing just trying to schedule appointments. Here, they were already done for us and all we had to do was show up! During these meetings, our goal was to explain the necessity of supporting the Medical Nutrition Equity Act. We shared our personal journey, then Rem shared his story and we spoke about the need for this bill. We shared information regarding the bill and those who have already signed on in support of it. We pushed to have them to back this initiative. Remington and I are just one small vessel used

Home Plate

in this situation. There are so many others who have made some powerful waves in this mission for insurance coverage. For them, we are grateful.

Remington's speech at the Congressional briefing session was both powerful and moving. When I looked around the room, I saw tears in the eyes of the listeners from Rem's honest words. He was able to connect and help them understand what it's like to live in his shoes, even if it's just for a moment.

We don't get nervous any longer with these meetings. We realize the importance of formula coverage for those whose lives depend on it, like Remington's. Congressmen are people just like we are, trying to make a difference. They want to fight for a purpose and feel that they're throwing their weight behind something important. We're just trying to convince them that our fight is the one they need to take on, sooner rather than later.

Of course, once we return home, we still have much follow up work to do. We'll send out thank you notes to those we met with and then follow up with emails and phone calls. Although we have accomplished a lot, there is still much work to be done at both the state and federal levels.

When Rem was first diagnosed, we never would have imagined that we'd be helping draft legislation. My thought was that somebody else does that sort of stuff. Now we are those somebodies, and we are in it for the long haul. Some legislation is passed quickly and others take years to pass. However long it takes, we are committed to getting this legislation passed on both the state and federal levels.

I believe we must have faith that our lives matter and that we'll make a difference. And no matter what, we must hold onto hope. Without hope, the world would be such an empty place."

I was really nervous about speaking in front of the Congressional staff, but I realized that I have a responsibility to help. My own situation has put me on the front lines. My mom told me once that we must be a voice for the voiceless. This is my way of being that voice.

Chapter 9:

Helping Others

Looking back over the years I struggled with my disease, I realized God had a plan for me. He allowed my struggles to make me strong so that I could use my experiences to help others. My parents taught me that we must make the path easier for those who follow. I don't know if I'm making it easier; all I'm trying to do is live each day, overcoming each obstacle in my way. When people see me, I hope they don't see a kid who can't eat. I hope they see an athlete. A son. A brother. A student. I hope they see someone determined to stay healthy. I hope they see someone who has overcome. Most of all, I hope they see resilience.

> *When people see me, I hope they don't see a kid who can't eat. I hope they see someone who has overcome. Most of all, I hope they see resilience.*

Home Plate

In May 2017, Neocate, the elemental formula manufacturer, asked me to do a video for them. While I was in New York for filming, I met a boy named Landon who has FPIES, Food Protein-Induced Entercolitis Syndrome—another type of disease that requires a formula diet. He's a cool kid who liked sports, so we hit it off right away. At the time, he had a handful of foods in his diet but also needed the formula as his nutritional source.

> *My parents had been constantly reminding me about being good to my body, but the bottom line was it was up to me.*

Several months later, Landon got really sick and had to switch to a formula-only diet. His mother reached out to mine and asked if I would consider talking to Landon. He was only ten at the time and I was a seventeen-year-old senior in high school, but I agreed to call and talk to him. I would FaceTime him in the afternoons and ask him how he was doing. There were times when it was awkward because I didn't know what to say. Even though we both loved sports, there was a vast age difference and Landon was also struggling with the big changes to his life and diet.

Helping Others

One afternoon, I opened up a little more about my own struggles. I told him that I knew how hard it was to switch to only formula when you're used to eating food. I reminded him that his body needed to get healthy and the only way was by drinking this stuff. I set a goal for him and promised I would send him a gift each time he reached a goal. I kept my promises, and Landon kept his, and eventually Landon was able to recover from that flare up.

I think I was able to get through to Landon because I understood too well what he was going through. When I was a sophomore, I was hungry all the time because of working out, the fact my body was growing, along with the normal cravings teenage boys get. There were times when I would sneak food and eat it just because I couldn't stand being hungry. When your diet is limited to nothing but liquid formula, sometimes you crave simply chewing. I would sneak snack crackers or cheese or whatever I could grab and eat on the sly. Of course, that meant I suffered coughing fits and constant sharp pains in my upper chest where my esophagus is located. I knew I was damaging my body and knew I should stop.

My parents started asking me questions because they knew I was sneaking food. They were really worried about the damage that I was doing to myself. In addi-

Home Plate

tion, my immune system weakened even more and I began catching every virus and cold imaginable, yet I continued to sneak food. At my endoscopy that summer, the doctor said my esophagus looked as bad as it had when I was first diagnosed. I had severe grooves and ridging and the tissue was inflamed. The doctor said that if I kept it up, my esophagus would lose its pliability and food would get stuck. Worse, I could lose my ability to swallow—forever. I knew what that meant—a feeding tube, which would change my life. No way, I decided. I needed to stop sneaking food. My parents had been constantly reminding me about being good to my body, but the bottom line was it was up to me. I had to fix it myself. No one else could. That was part of the message I gave to Landon, and maybe simply hearing that he was in control of how healthy he was—his choices would either make or break his health—perhaps that was what made a difference for him.

My parents have been instrumental in helping me to see the positive side of my situation, and to remember to look for ways to help others. I've also learned a lot from my other family members, like my Aunt Debbie. She's mentally handicapped but she loves soccer because of Dalton and baseball because of me. When she's at our games, she hollers "Dopey," for Dalton and "Rin Tin" for me. She's enthusiastic and self-assured, regardless of

Helping Others

her disabilities and the fact that she's missing a fingertip (another mentally handicapped student bit it off one day while she was at school). Aunt Debbie still smiles all the time and walks with her index finger up in the air like she's number one.

Her enthusiasm for life and her positive attitude are infectious. It encouraged me to work with special needs kids when I was in high school, as well as help out at the Special Olympics. Her zest for life stands as a reminder that we are all fortunate in some way, no matter what challenges we face.

I have learned a lot about family and teamwork from my coaches and teammates. My coaches have played a valuable role in teaching me the importance of being accountable to one another, and in helping mold me into a better player and a more responsible young man.

Over the years, I have also become involved with the student group at my church and through that, I met the high school pastor Chris Dotson. We have a lot in common and he has helped me grow in my faith and as a young man. He's become one of my best friends. I look to him as a brother and love him as a brother, too. I wouldn't be where I am today in my faith without Pastor Chris.

Home Plate

In the summer of 2017, I went on a mission trip to the Dominican Republic. That trip changed my whole outlook because I was reminded of how much we take for granted here in the U.S., like running water and air conditioning. We don't have to wait to pump our water before using it or rely on the breeze to cool us. The kids there play baseball on dirt fields with overgrown grass, rocks, and sometimes goats. Our fields are neatly manicured and maintained by the local parks and recreation department. If other kids only saw what it's like in the D.R., then they too would have a renewed sense of appreciation for all we have been blessed with here.

> *I've been very fortunate that my family and extended family have also taught me a lot about faith.*

The Dominicans are an incredible, passionate group of people. Not just about baseball but also about each other. They welcome and embrace anyone and were excited to play our baseball team. Their entire approach to life is so different from ours in the U.S. Here, it seems we're always rushing around about things that are meaningless or don't make a difference: Trying to beat that red light, or not being late for lunch with friends. In the Dominican Republic, they take time to talk, shake someone's hand, and they travel a bit

Helping Others

slower. They don't have the technology we do there so being there is like traveling back in time. Kids are all outside playing with one another instead of stuck inside the house playing video games. For many of these kids, their only escape is being outside playing baseball and dreaming that they're the next ones called up to the major leagues.

In the summer of 2018, I went on a mission trip to a small town in northern England. While we were there, we hosted sports camps for kids who ranged in age from elementary to high school. We split into different teams based on the countries that participated in the recent World Cup. We played soccer, volleyball, tag, dodgeball, and capture the flag. In the middle of the day, we took a break and sat down for a lesson about Jesus from the team leaders. My favorite part of the trip was the relationships the other team leaders and I built with the kids. There were so many meaningful and memorable moments in that trip.

The only obstacles I've encountered as I go on these international trips is how to ship my shakes over ahead of time and how many I should bring with me. All of that pales in comparison when I see what other kids go through in areas much poorer than here.

Home Plate

I've been very fortunate that my family and extended family have also taught me a lot about faith. For a time, my dad was sick. I was scared because my dad is my best friend. We do everything together. Our afternoons were spent with him throwing to me for batting practice and hitting ground balls so I can work on my ball-handling skills. We also spent a lot of time just talking. My dad ended up having major surgery. My mother stayed at the hospital and my older brother was at his own house, so I spent a week with my buddy Max and his family. I remember one night after we'd returned to their home after a game, Ms. Mary, Max's mom, came up and gave me a much-needed hug. Suddenly, I didn't feel so alone in my worries. I kept praying that everything would be all right and it eventually was.

Just before Christmas in 2017, my parents asked me to come into the TV room to talk with them. I figured this had to be some pretty serious stuff—and it was. My mother had just been diagnosed with breast cancer. I remember thinking how unfair that was, that our family had been through enough already. That night I cried and prayed.

 That Christmas, I was diagnosed with breast cancer. My first thought was, I'm not going to spoil the holidays and then my next thought was, This is Remington's senior year. I don't want to

take away from it. I wasn't sure how I was going to share this news with our boys. I held onto the hope that I would be healed. Mike was a pillar of support and encouragement as were Dalton and Remington.

After coming home from an appointment one day, I told my boys that I wanted them to hug me for as long as it took me to take three long deep breaths. I didn't want to let them go so quickly anymore, and held on until those three long breaths were over. It became our "thing" every time I hugged them. Sometimes, one of them would say, "Hurry up and breathe already!" but they never let go.

When I was recovering from my lumpectomy, Remington helped me do my arm exercises and every time I was ready to quit, he'd urge, "Just one more, mom. C'mon you can do it." My son was telling me the very same motivational words he'd say to himself so he wouldn't give up.

Jesus blessed me with His healing and I am eternally grateful."

It took time and medical intervention, but my mother's cancer is now in remission. Despite all that our family has gone through, I firmly believe God has a plan and that He put us here, in this exact position, to help others. Our family works hard not to allow negativity to drag us down. Most of all, we have each other's backs and when any one of us needs help or just a hug, we're there for each other. I wouldn't wish EoE on anyone, but I do wish that anyone who is struggling with a challenging illness has a family like mine to make their journey easier.

Chapter 10:

A Note from Dad

From the minute you learn your child has a medical condition, you wonder what life will be like. Will they be able to enjoy the same activities as a "normal" kid? Will they miss out on life? I worried about all that and more the day we got Remington's diagnosis. As a father of two boys, I wanted Remington to be able to enjoy the same experiences as his older brother.

From the minute you learn your child has a medical condition, you wonder what life will be like.

A friend of mine, Darrin, told me about his family's annual hunting trip. When I was younger, my family and I went camping, which created some of my fondest memories. When we had the boys, I wanted to start some kind of yearly tradition with them. But hunting?

Home Plate

Having a child with an illness that didn't allow him to eat was hard enough; thinking about hunting with both my boys was difficult to embrace at first. I thought of the camaraderie that Darrin and his family shared every year, so when his dad, Wayne, asked me if I'd like to come. I decided to tag along to get an idea of what their trip entailed. Wayne and Darrin treated us like family from then on and our families have been hunting together ever since.

My oldest son, Dalton, didn't care for hunting as much as he enjoyed riding the four wheelers in the camp. On our first hunt together, he was ready to leave the stand and go riding by 7:30 am. He had very little interest in the hunting aspect but enjoyed participating in the work weekends so he could ride the four wheelers. I remember Wayne laughing, "That 'Rooster' (referring to Dalton) is going to scare off all the deer with all that noise he's making."

When it came to introducing Remington to hunting, I was really afraid he wouldn't enjoy it. Remington couldn't eat, so when I told him I wanted to take him hunting, he asked, "Why am I going if I can't eat the meat we get?" The boys knew that whatever game was shot was to be eaten, so my reply was simple and to the point. "Because you will be helping the family by providing food for us."

A Note from Dad

That first weekend hunt, Remington was nine years old. We didn't see anything to shoot, which was totally fine with me and Rem. He had a passion for being in the woods. He loved sitting around the campfire at night and telling stories, laughing, and cutting up. Shooting contests, scouting the woods, and just seeing nature in all its beauty proved to be good therapy for Remington.

> At that point I realized that this ten-year-old, who had not eaten food in six years, understood the rest of the family needed to eat to survive.

To my amazement, by the second year he seemed like a seasoned hunter. We'd start before sunup, then come out of the woods around 10:30 am and meet back in camp. We'd have lunch, I'd eat a sandwich or a hot dog and he'd drink his formula, then rest or prep for the evening hunt. Remington wanted to sit and stay in the woods longer than anyone. We would be the last two to come back in the morning and first to go out in the evening. This dedication paid off on an evening hunt when Remington was ten-years-old.

A deer walked out into the field early one evening. Remington was so nervous that it was hard for me not to laugh. "Buck fever" had struck my young boy. He was shaking and breathing hard. The kid made so much noise I couldn't believe the deer stayed there instead of scampering away.

When Remington raised his rifle, the stock bumped against the window jam and his feet banged the bottom of the blind. Thank God the deer stayed in the food plot and Remington was able to harvest his first buck. The two of us were so excited we missed our high five. We called home so he could tell mom about his first deer. Remington was shaking to the point of not being able to hold the phone. His voice trembled and tears of joy ran down his cheeks. "Mom, I got meat for the family!" he shouted.

At that point I realized that this ten-year-old, who had not eaten food in six years, understood the rest of the family needed to eat to survive. The emotions running through me were overwhelming. I was so proud of him, not just for the harvest but for his understanding and joy to help his family.

Over the years, Remington and I have been on many hunts together and I believe the experience has brought us closer. Through our trips, we have been able to share different emotions and experiences. As parents, Stephanie and I live with this illness as well as his brother, Dalton, but not in the way Remington

A Note from Dad

has had to. I've told him many times, "I see you living with this every day but I can't imagine what it's like to walk in your shoes."

And I really can't. I live in a world where I can eat pretty much whatever I want, whenever I want. I can smell a hamburger and know that I can have one for dinner that night, if I choose. Remington doesn't have that same luxury, so every run to McDonald's that his friends make or every pizza they order at a party is something he can't have. We have watched him endure endless tests and painful food trials, and through it all, his same strong, irrepressible spirit has endured. As parents, we can only guide our children to the best of our ability and knowledge. We are going to make mistakes. That is a part of life; failure is required in order to grow as a person.

From the minute he was diagnosed, we have always told Remington, "The world doesn't care that you can't eat," so that has never been a focus of his upbringing. We focus on what he can control and not what others think. The early years were hard, really hard. A lot of anger, depression, hate, and sadness were a part of our lives. Through countless hours of counseling, activities, and time spent camping we learned how to navigate through the hard times.

Home Plate

His athleticism guided us to baseball—the one sport where he didn't exert too much energy and learned to focus on team building. This structure was important for him, both physically and mentally. When he was in eighth grade he played soccer. He wanted to try the sport his brother loved and excelled at. He did well, but we discovered he had lost around ten pounds in a span of six weeks and that was too much. It took a little over a year for him to gain that weight back. Tennis was also too much running. Basketball, the same. Golf was definitely out of the question because he lacked the patience for it.

He fell in love with the game of baseball and worked hard at it because he found he could control how well he played, unlike his disease. However, the early years were hard as he learned the sport and developed his skills.

We put a batting cage in the back yard, and every day after work I'd go out there and pitch to him for batting practice. The hours we spent correcting and molding his confidence proved worthwhile for his positive mental ability. In addition to the daily batting practices, we would routinely throw in the yard to strengthen his arm. During all this practice, we talked—about his day, about what he was going through, and about what worried and stressed him. We taught Remington that failure was okay and that one must have a short memory for any mistakes. There were days when that was a challenging task, espe-

A Note from Dad

cially when our kid tried to prove he wasn't really any different than the other kids on that ball field.

I reminded him many times to move on and forget what happened, to have a short memory, like when he struck out or missed a throw. Sometimes the other players are better than you, and maybe next time it will be your turn to be the better player. As Cal Ripken Jr. has stated, "Baseball is a game of failure in many ways. As a hitter, you fail seven out of ten times, so you have to figure out how to deal with failure." The game will certainly keep you humble.

If not for baseball, we truly believe Remington would be a completely different person. Baseball gave Rem the ability to set goals for himself and learn how to improve upon his mistakes. Most importantly, baseball gave him a responsibility to others on his team. It helped him with accountability. Being part of a team taught him that it takes hard work to succeed and that he shouldn't quit on his team or on life.

When Remington moved onto high school, we added trips to baseball stadiums as part of our bonding time. One year we went to St. Louis to see the Cardinals play. There were a few humps to navigate around, such as Rem having enough formula for the trip and finding a hotel near the stadium so the formula would be close by

Home Plate

when he needed more. We found the perfect hotel overlooking the stadium and for that sunny afternoon, we were just like any other father and son.

Remington's resilience has inspired us—his mom, his brother Dalton and me—more than I could have imagined.

I admire my son greatly. He has this ability to go through life without eating with a strength I'm not sure I would have had if put into his same situation. He is determined and focused, and Rem has a drive like no one I've ever met. He has two phrases that say everything about how strong he is: "You were meant to push the standards not accept them." And "Achieve everything they said you never would."

In addition, I find that I turn to some of the motivational quotes he uses whenever I need a boost:

"It's not who you are that holds you back, it's who you think you're not." — Eric Thomas

"I go harder because I know where I was at and I know where I want to go…" —Deshaun Watson

A Note from Dad

"It's what you practice in private that you will be rewarded for in public."—Tony Robbins

There have been periods in our lives when I have questioned God as to why us? I remember a time when I turned my back on God because I felt He did the same to me and my family. I have prayed repeatedly for God to heal my son, and in times of desperation I would cry out wanting to know why Rem hadn't been healed yet.

One day, a guy I work with gave me a book he had purchased at his church. He said he was thinking about me and thought I might like it. At that moment, I realized God had not turned against me. He wanted me to seek His guidance, now more than ever. He'd given me that message from my coworker and that book to remind me to look to Him—always. I needed His help for the greater good, not just for Remington but for my entire family.

Remington's resilience has inspired us—his mom, his brother Dalton and me—more than I could have imagined. Instead of wanting to know why we were being punished because he had EoE, I now realize God could not have blessed us more by entrusting Remington to our family. Throughout our journey, God has carried us and will continue to carry us in the days to come.

From Dalton Walls:

 I don't remember a whole lot about when we first knew something was wrong with Rem because I was only around eight or nine-years-old. What I do remember is that Rem would always throw up at the dinner table and I didn't want to eat while he was sitting there. We couldn't figure out why this was happening or what we could do. Eventually, my parents found a doctor who was able to identify what was wrong with him.

After that, my parents said we wouldn't be eating dinner together anymore, which was cool for me because it meant I was able to eat in front of the TV every night. They also said we would only go out to dinner on birthdays. Other than that, life was the same.

In some ways, life was the same, but in others it wasn't, I realize as I look back now. There was so much that changed. We stopped socializing with people and really didn't do many fun things any more. Our vacations were spent around Rem's hospital visits. This was a tough time for all of us, mostly because we were trying to adjust to something that we didn't even understand. I know that my parents did the best they could and they have apologized to Rem and I both for mistakes made along the way. To be honest, those early years, life was anything but easy.

A lot of people hear about his condition and figure we have to treat him differently, but we don't. He and I had the same love/hate relationship that any other brothers have. I coached his soccer team for the two years he played which was a really great experience, and I loved going to his high school baseball games. He does everything like a normal person—honestly, I haven't thought about his inability to eat in at least a few years because we just don't see him that way. He's perfectly capable of doing anything he wants in life and I couldn't be a prouder older brother of the man he's starting to become."

> We choose to find a deeper purpose and try to focus on the positive outcomes. Life is truly worth living.

Home Plate

Chapter 11:

How to Truly Live

by Mom

Your family might not be dealing with EoE, but you may have a child with asthma or a severe allergy or diabetes, or any of the thousands of things that can make them "different". It's important for your child to have a positive, accepting environment in school and at home. Having that environment starts with you, as a parent, and the example you set. Don't be afraid to seek outside counseling. Sometimes, it helps to have someone outside of your family facilitate communication through the concerns, hurts, and struggles a new diagnosis may bring. Additionally, if you're unsure of the medical diagnosis, then seek another opinion. Spend time researching the new information so you can ask the doctor questions to help in your

These are the ways we teach our children to cope with the good and the not-so-good, as well as how to self-advocate.

own understanding and in helping your child understand as well.

It's important to have a doctor who is willing to take the time to guide you and give you direction on how to properly care for your child. If they don't have the time to help you, then find another doctor who will take the time. We've been blessed to have crossed paths with some passionate doctors along the way, from Remington's pediatrician to his GI doctors to his orthopedic surgeon.

Throughout this journey, our family has developed more of an appreciation for life. I think many families that face major health issues can relate. We choose to find a deeper purpose and try to focus on the positive outcomes. Life is truly worth living.

At School:

When your child is ready for school, there may be one or several people who will need to be involved in their transitioning into school, such as the school nurse, guidance counselor, principal or assistant principal, school or county psychologist, and the teacher(s). Meet with all of those people and make sure they are briefed on and understand your child's needs.

How to Truly Live

During that meeting, provide an abbreviated version of your child's disease. Avoid giving a long, detailed history. Instead, focus the discussion on how your child's needs might impact the classroom and how to meet them without disrupting the learning environment. Try to leave your emotions aside and focus on the task at hand. When we allow our emotions to take over, we often lose the opportunity to make the connections necessary for the success of our children. Kids don't want to stand out, therefore give the school staff options to maintain as much normalcy as possible. For us, instead of having Rem drink his "shake" elsewhere, we asked if he could drink it in the classroom since we didn't want him missing any of the material. Eventually, his shakes became the norm in the classroom and kids stopped noticing.

Talk with the school nurse and guidance counselor about a care plan that states your child's health needs and have those staff members educate the other adults who will be around your child during the day. We showed the administration the product Rem would be drinking so they would know when they saw a kid with an orange-colored juice box that this was a necessity for Rem, not an option.

Every year that Remington was in elementary school, I went into the classroom to educate his classmates. The nurse, administrators, and guidance counselors made themselves available to come in for a half-hour presentation. I invited his classmates' parents as well. My goal was to educate as many people about the disease as I could. I would show the "Just a Glimpse" video from APFED and then answer any questions.

In my talk, I explained that Rem could still participate in celebrations and treat giveaways but he couldn't eat any of the goodies. He could only drink his "shake" and water. By explaining what food does to his body, the kids were better able to understand and accept him. It also provided reasoning why Rem would need to drink his shake during class time and not just during lunch. That way, he wasn't perceived as receiving special privileges. When classmates feel that others are receiving favoritism, it creates tension. Students want to feel that they're all being treated equally, so explaining "the why behind the what" helped the other children understand this was a necessity, not a privilege.

Before school starts, I recommend sitting down with your child and openly communicating the day-to-day procedures your child will experience. Run through their school schedule and talk about when it might be a good time to drink that shake or go to the clinic for their medicine. Check in with your child often throughout the school year and ask them how things

Most of all, love your child. Your child is a gift from God—to you and to the world.

are going. We did this daily in the first few weeks of every school year. What things are working well? What things aren't? How is your child feeling throughout the day? Talk about the pitfalls of the day, too. Have your child share what didn't work that day and ask why. Then, together, come up with a plan to make it better. These are the ways we teach our children to cope with the good and the not-so-good, as well as how to self-advocate.

The ultimate goal is for your child to grow socially and learn while in school. If you put the disease as the focus while they're in school, making them stand out as the "sick child", your child will find it hard to be accepted by his or her peers. Friends are an important aspect of any child's day and making it easier for other kids to understand and accept your child helps kids create bonds in the classroom. Building relationships with peers and teachers is essential for a child to succeed later in life.

Home Plate

At home:

Remain hopeful at home. Find a phrase that will spark humor and encourage your child to move forward. They will have bad days, just like us. Remind your child, and yourself, that everything we walk through today prepares us for tomorrow. We must inspire our children to have courage. Pastor Ken Whitten once said in a Sunday message, "Courage isn't the absence of fear; it's the moving forward in spite of fear." Our children must have the courage to conquer life.

Remind your child that he or she can do anything regardless of their circumstances. Our children are already stronger because they have to overcome and endure so much more than others. In knowing that, they are already one step closer to greatness!

Expect your child to attend school. If he or she is not able to attend, then arrange for education to take place at home. Expect your child to do well in school and don't allow their circumstance to lower the bar. There were many times when we had to remind Remington that he still had to go to school and work hard. His medical condition wasn't an excuse to do poorly.

Engage your child in outside activities, such as sports, art, dance, drama, etc. These activities help build confi-

How to Truly Live

dence and teach our children to make friends based on something they have in common. Putting Remington in art class allowed him to express his feelings. Putting him in baseball helped him find his passion and strength.

Tell your child that he or she is awesome and remind yourself of that, too. Life is truly a blessing and we have all been chosen to make a difference. The grace and strength that they have in the face of whatever obstacle they encounter will be a lesson to those around them.

Most of all, love your child. Love them when they struggle or when they succeed. Love them when they are brave, or when they are weak, and love them when they are strong. Love them and hug them and accept them for all that they are, and all that God made them to be. Your child is a gift from God—to you and to the world.

HOW TO LIVE WITH SOMETHING NO ONE UNDERSTANDS - by Remington

Over the years, I have taken several phrases to heart, and pull them out whenever things get tough:

> *It is what it is.*

> *Change your mindset and see your circumstances as something you're going to overcome.*

> *You are more powerful than anything life throws at you.*

> *If you don't have faith and don't believe in yourself, you're done—you've already lost.*

> *Nobody is going to come and live your life for you, nobody is going to come and take your pain away from you. You need to figure out how to get past it and then stay on track.*

As Eric Thomas said, "You have to use your pain to push you to where you want to go."

Maybe you're struggling right now and wondering how to find that life you always dreamed you'd have. Start by viewing yourself differently. I don't see myself as sick. I see myself as *capable*. Yeah, I get down, especially when my body rejects a new food and I get really sick from a food trial. It can take days, sometimes weeks, to get well again but I still push through. I still go to school, to baseball practice, and to my workouts. Doing all of that is a choice I make. Make the choice to push through when things are tough.

Google motivational speakers and start listening to them and find one or two who motivate and encourage you. Let their words be yours until you find your own. Let them fuel you to work harder. You'll be amazed at the sense of accomplishment you'll feel when you start doing better in school, start working out, or begin improving on something you already know how to do. No one can take that accomplishment from you.

Remember, today is only one day. You might be struggling right now, but tomorrow will come and it will be better. Whatever you do, don't feel sorry for yourself. Remove yourself from negative people because they will bring you down. You already have a lot on your plate so it's necessary to surround yourself with positive people who will lift you up on your darker days.

Help others. I did this by being the leader on my baseball team, offering encouragement to my teammates with a word or comment. I also did it on my mission trips. You can't feel sorry for yourself when you see someone else who has absolutely nothing yet manages to smile and laugh.

Having faith is powerful. Faith is believing in something you don't see and gaining strength from that. My faith is in God, knowing that He's with me every step of the way on my journey. I thank Chris and Kelly for their lessons on that. I remember a time when I was in so much pain from my disease. One night, I cried and cried in the shower, pleading with God to help me. To heal me. I came out of that shower so depleted I didn't feel the pain anymore. I was so exhausted that I went to bed and slept deeply that night. The next morning was another day and I felt a little better. The pain wasn't all gone, but I discovered I could deal with it better. God had heard me, and answered my prayer by giving me rest and a brighter day in the morning.

I know that one day I will be healed. It's just not time for that yet. Until then, I am going to live my life to the fullest and keep looking forward to what's ahead of me.

Chapter 12:

An Update from the Walls Family

The years that have been since we first started writing this book have been filled with changes and new opportunities. We have been blessed and challenged, but through it all, our family keeps fighting.

From Stephanie:

One of our biggest adjustments was Remington graduating high school and going off to college. That experience was definitely a transition for both Rem

God pointed me to the people who would help and my faith guided us the rest of the way to the finish line.

and us. Moving any child to college is an adjustment but moving him out of state to a college where he knew nobody and no one knew about his disease was a huge change for everyone. His first year away from home he spent living in a college dorm. As parents, we wanted him to experience the true college life.

For Rem, such a common thing wasn't as simple as it might be for other students. Because Rem has a medical 504 plan, we met with the housing coordinator to discuss the need for a larger refrigerator and the need to be exempted from the required food plan. We wanted to make sure the college knew what he needed. The day we moved him into the dorm, he was both excited and nervous about losing the safety net of his small hometown. As we drove home, Mike and I had to let go and trust God, and most of all, trust in the verse of Jeremiah 29:11.

Once a month, we load up his cases of nutrition and haul them up to him. Rem has a wagon that he uses to transport his shakes to his dorm room. He's grown accustomed to the inevitable questions and the routine.

The first semester was tough for him. He hadn't met too many people and wasn't comfortable being out of his element. There were times when Rem would call to say he was coming home because he was struggling. Instead, we went up to visit him, so he could stay on campus instead of coming home when things got tough. Rem was still struggling with missing his friends back home,

An Update from the Walls Family

and with not having the same comfortable acceptance that he was used to. On one of our visits, we went to the parents' lunch and met other parents as well as the dean of the college for new students. On Sunday morning, we attended a local church as a family, and introduced Rem to several people. After the sermon, Rem was inspired to drive up to the baseball fields that Sunday afternoon. Surprisingly, the coach was there and Rem talked to him about how much he missed baseball and how he wanted to be more connected with the college. Rem became the coach's assistant and that opened many more doors to meet people who were like-minded. Many of those guys have become good, lifelong friends.

As he grew more comfortable on campus, Rem began to open up to others about why he needed to drink formula. He found out the easiest thing to say was just "Google me". Then they could read up on his story and come back later with questions.

Before Rem's sophomore year we moved him into an apartment with a baseball buddy named Jordan. What a gift that was to have such a trusted influence from a similar family as his roommate. Rem's sophomore year flew by and he moved away from baseball to begin working and earning money. He had to learn to balance this new responsibility, but he has definitely made it work.

Home Plate

Throughout this transition, Rem worked alongside me on making changes in the Florida legislation. Whenever I needed him to, he would drive from Georgia to Tallahassee to meet with lawmakers to pursue the need for the bill to cover medical formula for people who needed it. Rem spoke in front of the various committees and would meet one on one with legislators to convince them of the need to champion this initiative. It was a lot to ask of a college student but Rem continued pursuing this because of his conviction that it's the right thing to do to help people.

After three years of working on this, the legislation was finally signed into law! Now the State of Florida has coverage for those in need of medical formula, but right now, only for those who are on the state's medical insurance. There is still work to do on the insurance front, something we will continue pursuing in the future. When I look back on this journey, I realize that God guided me through it every step of the way. I had no idea what I was doing. I just had a passion for doing what was right for others that followed us. God pointed me to the people who would help and my faith guided us the rest of the way to the finish line.

Overall, college life has been a blessing for Rem and for us as well. It has offered Rem the opportunity to grow up and branch out while learning to make adjustments

An Update from the Walls Family

to his life. College life forced me to let go and trust that God had it all under control.

Although…there was that one time when Rem smashed his finger with weights and my mom instincts kicked in. The gym called an ambulance just to be safe, but the paramedics said all he needed was stitches. I wanted to get in the car right then and drive up there to help, but Mike said we had to let him figure this out on his own, which we did. He's an adult now, and like any parent, I struggle with that change, but he's turning into a wonderful, compassionate, and gracious young man, and we couldn't be prouder of him.

From Remington:

I remember the day I packed up my truck and drove away from home, heading for college and a whole new period of my life. I loved moving into my first dorm and living on my own. I had a lot of fun setting up my dorm room and organizing everything I needed.

But after my parents drove away and I was on my own, I realized I had no friends here and that I had to force myself to meet people. Here's the strange thing: most people make acquaintances when they gather at the cafeteria or restaurants, but since I had no need to have a meal plan, meeting at the on-campus cafeteria wasn't an option for me. I found myself going to class and not really meeting people. Between classes, I'd hide myself away in my dorm.

I was having a hard time adjusting to my first semester away from home. I called home often, and every time I mentioned coming home, my parents discouraged me from doing that. They wanted me to stay and adjust, but it was tough. When my parents came up for the parents' weekend, they signed us up to do every one of the activities, and included me in every connection they made. I felt like the odd man out. Here I was hanging out with my parents at all the campus activities and I really hadn't made any friends yet.

It wasn't until my parents took me to church one Sunday morning that things began to turn around. The sermon that day empowered me to get out and take a chance. The pastor played a video of a runner who pulls a hamstring while running a race. Instead of giving up, he chose to force himself across the finish line so it would show on his race record that he did finish the race, which was an almost impossible feat with his injury. The runner's father came down the stands and helped his son walk to the finish line. The pastor told

An Update from the Walls Family

us this is what God does in our lives—He carries us if we let him.

When my parents left to go home, I found myself wanting to make a change in my life, one that was the opposite of giving up, so I got in my truck and drove to the ballfields in hopes of talking to the coach. I couldn't believe that he was there on a Sunday but he was. During our conversation, I shared that I had played baseball my whole life and was interested in trying out but in the meantime I wanted to do something with the team. He agreed to let me be the team's manager. That moment changed everything for me.

The connection with the baseball team helped me make connections with players and made me feel like I had a real purpose again. When I wasn't in class, I was with the team. Later, I tried out for the team but didn't make it because the coach said I was too small and that I needed to gain weight. Was I disappointed? Yeah but I've been disappointed before so I didn't let it get me down. I was just glad to be a part of a family again.

During that first year, I missed my family, friends and just the comfortable part of people knowing me and my situation. When I moved to college, no one knew anything about me and my EoE, and now it was up to

Home Plate

me to explain it. In the beginning I felt weird about bringing a lunchbox with my shakes because no one on the team knew me. But when my new friends asked, I found myself just telling them to Google me. Sometimes, they'd do it right then and there and then ask questions.

Find your faith, dig deep, and you'll reach that next step!

The second semester was easier with the friendships I made on the team, but then our Florida legislation kicked in gear and I was having to drive back and forth to the Florida capitol to speak before the different legislative committees. It was difficult to balance everything with the legislation, school, and my team responsibilities which meant for a rough semester academically. I was busy writing speeches, practicing the key points I wanted to make, because this year was different, and the stakes were higher. We had finally found a representative on the House side to take up our cause and unite with Senator Stargel on the Senate side.

When our bill made it onto the calendar for committee, we had to drop everything to get there in time to present our case. I remember the first time my name was called. I was nervous. I stood up and walked to the podium that faced the legislators on the committee. The senator who sponsored our bill was seated next to the podium and she shared information about the bill and about me and my situation of not having insurance cover my medical formula. Then it was my turn to speak.

I remember speaking from my heart about what it's like for a kid with EoE. How we can't just grab food whenever, how we need to carry formula everywhere we go. I used one of my shakes as a visual aid to drive home the point. I told them I was in college to make a better life for my future and that I didn't want to live off the system just because my medical formula is too expensive. Most of all, I told them that I've been taught to stand up for what is right and that I feel I have a responsibility to be the voice for others who are like me.

I was so nervous leading up to this first speech, but I found that I was naturally comfortable sharing the need for this coverage because it's the right thing to do. We made several trips to Tallahassee to testify, and people began to recognize us in the halls. Once in a while a legislator would say, "Great job on your speech."

After my mom and I had exhausted every avenue we could think of, we found out that our bill wasn't moving on to the next committee in the house, which meant we'd have to start all over again next year. We'd have to start over again finding support and sponsors and writing bill language.

Our Senator said she was looking into other options, but my mom kept working hard on the bill language with her to make it cover as many people as possible. Then on a Friday night in April, my mom called to say that the bill had passed!

I can't describe the feelings I felt because there was so much wrapped up in it—from the thought of all the time and effort we put in to make this happen, to the knowledge that other people were going to get the formula they need to survive. This was huge!

As wonderful as the passage of the law was, it still only helps a fraction of the people who need the formula because it only covers people who carry State of Florida insurance. The way the law is now, I am still unable to receive coverage for my medical formula. We're still fighting to get a bill passed that will require insurance companies to cover it.

I have learned so much in the past few years, especially that in order to succeed, you have to fail. I learned to take risks, to handle things on my own, and to face the things I was afraid of. I have learned that I can make a difference, if I stand up and use my voice.

We were invited to go to Jacksonville to Governor DeSantis's on-site location to watch the bill being signed. It was amazing to be standing beside him, hear him mention our names and applaud our efforts. He gave us the pen that he used to sign it, and suddenly, the bill was real.

Since writing the first edition of this book, I've had several opportunities to share my story of perseverance and how through it all, God has been with me. God has been the driving force for my life. I want to inspire other kids to not give up when they face a tough situation. The easiest thing to do is quit. But to stay at it and push through the hard times—now that makes you stronger. Find your faith, dig deep, and you'll reach that next step!

Home Plate

Resources

If someone in your family is suffering from EoE or any kind of GI condition, here are some resources that helped us:

Organizations:

American Partnership for Eosinophilic Disorders (APFED)
Passionately embraces, supports, and improves the lives of patients and families affected by eosinophil-associated diseases through education and awareness, research, support, and advocacy.
1-713-493-7719
https://apfed.org

Inspire/Health and Wellness Support Groups and Communities
Connects patients, families, friends, caregivers and health professionals for health and wellness support.
https://www.inspire.com

Nutricia – Neocate
Amino Acid Formula
1-800-365-7354
https://www.neocate.com
https://www.neocate.com/food-allergy-conditions-symptoms/eosinophilic-esophagitis/

Cincinnati Children's Hospital Medical Center
Cincinnati Center for Eosinophilic Disorders
3333 Burnet Avenue
Cincinnati, OH 45229
513-636-2233
www.cincinnatichildrens.org/service/c/eosinophilic-disorders

CURED Foundation
Campaign Urging Research for Eosinophilic Disorders
CURED is a not-for-profit foundation dedicated to those suffering from Eosinophilic Gastrointestinal Diseases (EGID), including eosinophilic esophagitis (EoE), eosinophilic gastritis (EG), eosinophilic colitis (EC) and other eosinophilic disorders.
www.curedfoundation.org

Food Protein-Induced Enterocolitis Syndrome (FPIES) Foundation
P.O. Box 304
Stewartville, MN 55976
www.fpiesfoundation.org

National Organization for Rare Disorders (NORD)
National Headquarters, CT Office
55 Kenosia Avenue
Danbury, CT 06810
Phone: 203-744-0100
Fax: 203-263-9938
https://rarediseases.org

Genetic and Rare Diseases (GARD) Information Center
PO Box 8126
Gaithersburg, MD 20898-8126
1-301-251-4925
1-888-205-2311
http://rarediseases.info.nih.gov/GARD

Books:

Chronic Kids, Constant Hope by Elizabeth Hoekstra and Mary Bradford

5 Love Languages by Gary Chapman
http://www.5lovelanguages.com/gary-chapman/

Awaken the Giant Within by Tony Robbins
Unlimited Power by Tony Robbins

Motivational Speakers:

Home Plate

Eric Thomas
https://www.etinspires.com

Tony Robbins
https://www.tonyrobbins.com

About the Authors

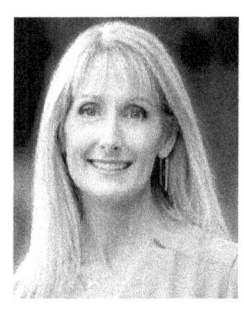

Stephanie Walls

Stephanie is blessed with a loving husband, Mike and their two sons, Dalton and Remington and their dogs, Sadie and Hank Aaron. She has taught middle school English for seventeen years after changing careers to have the same schedule as her children. She has an infectious laugh and her friends call her "Miss Sunshine." She has dedicated her time to giving back to help others along the way. Currently, she is pursuing legislation both federally and statewide that will help make a difference in the lives of others. She is guided by her belief in hope and grounded by her faith. She's just an ordinary person trying to make an extraordinary difference.

Home Plate

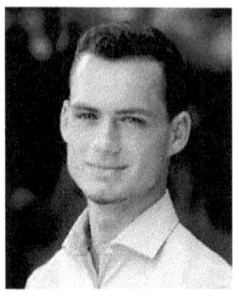

Remington Walls

Remington is in college at Valdosta State University. He has a passion for baseball. He has overcome immense odds throughout his life to be a positive role model to others. He is pursuing legislative efforts alongside his mother at the state and federal levels to help make a change. He believes that everyone has challenges but it's how one chooses to face those challenges that determines one's strength and purpose.

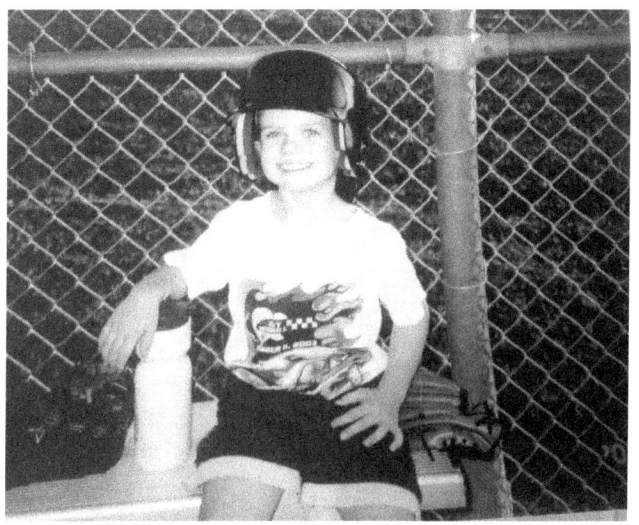

Rem, 4, ready for baseball practice

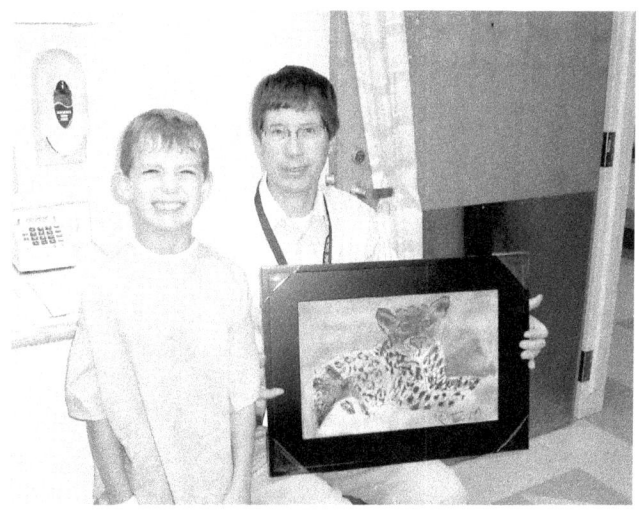

Rem giving his art work to Dr. Putnam

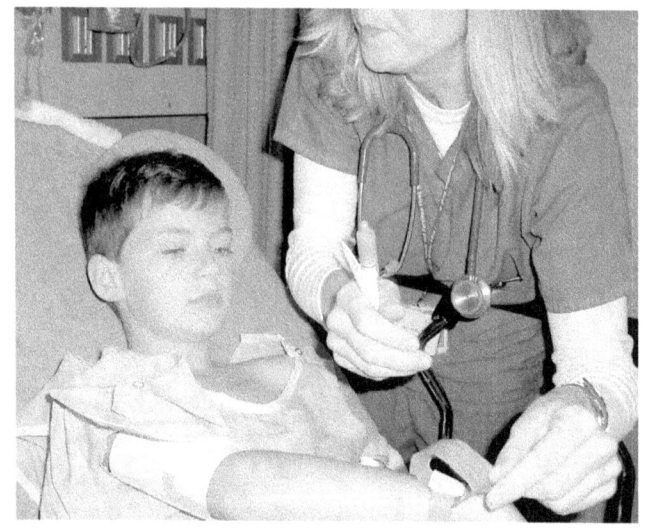

Rem, 6, at CCHMC for another endoscopy

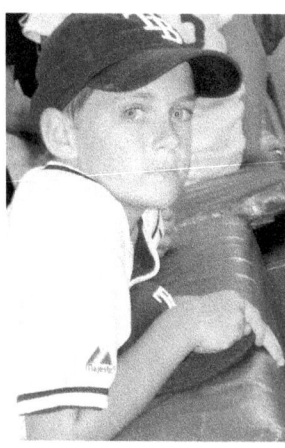

Rem, 6, at Rays Baseball game

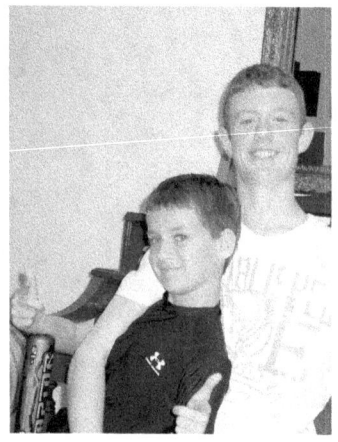

Rem, fourth grade, with brother Dalton

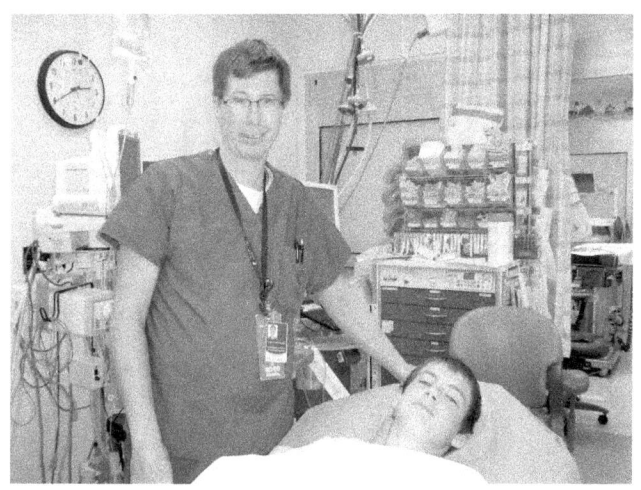

Dr. Putnam with Rem, 12, at CCHMC for another endoscopy

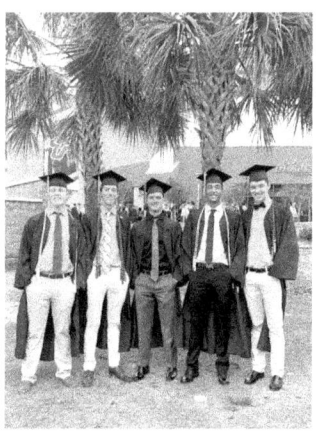

2018 LOL High School Graduation with best buds; Matt Geiger, Dave Puhalski, Remington (center), Edgar Vasquez and Ethan Terliamis

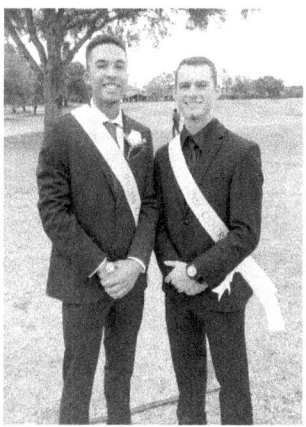

Edgar Vasquez with Rem for 2018 LOLHS Prom Court representatives

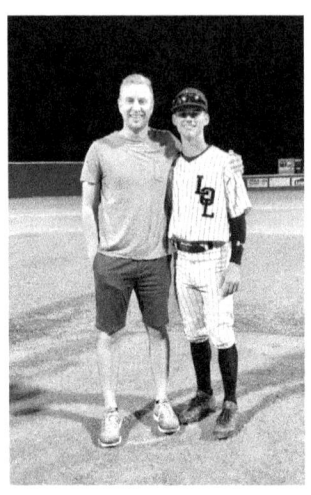
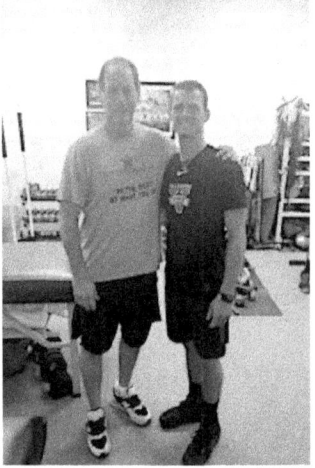

Pastor Chris Dotson with Rem at LOLHS Baseball Senior Night 2018

Trainer Larry Mayol with Rem

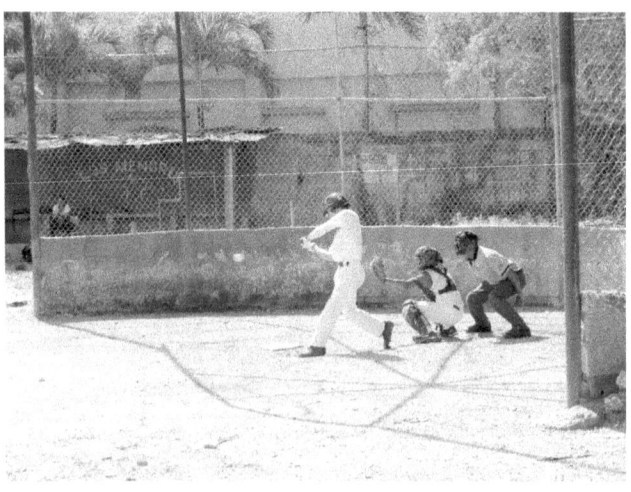

Rem in the Dominican Republic - July 2017

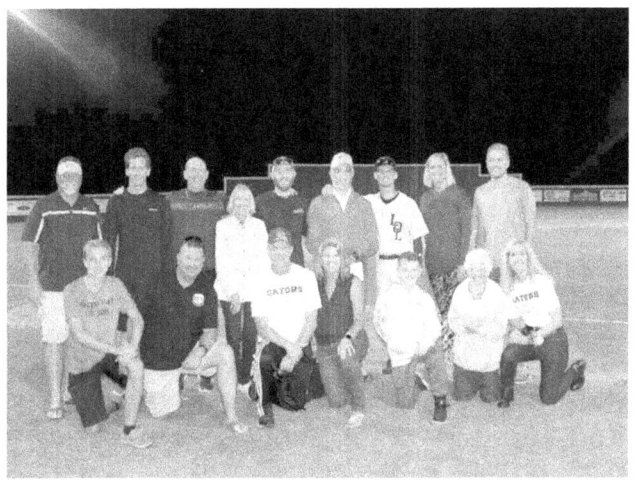

Rem's family at LOLHS Baseball Senior Night 2018 (back row standing from left to right is Uncle Ron, Samuel, Uncle Steve, Grandma, Dalton, Papa, Rem, Aunt Chrissy, Pastor Chris. Front row kneeling from left to right is Owen, Uncle Jeff, dad, Aunt Cissy, Drew, Aunt Debbie and mom

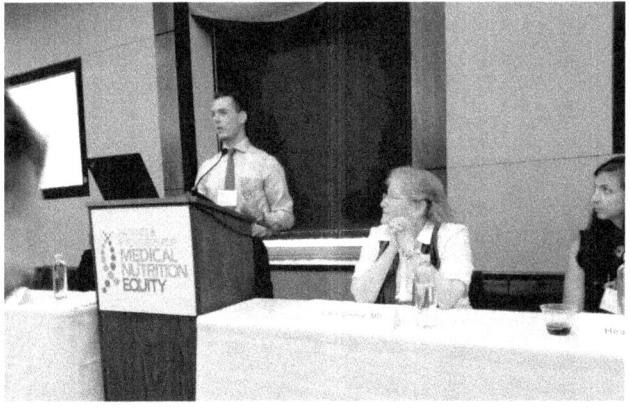

Rem speaking at congressional briefing session, Capitol Hill, for support of the Medical Nutrition Equity Act, June 2018

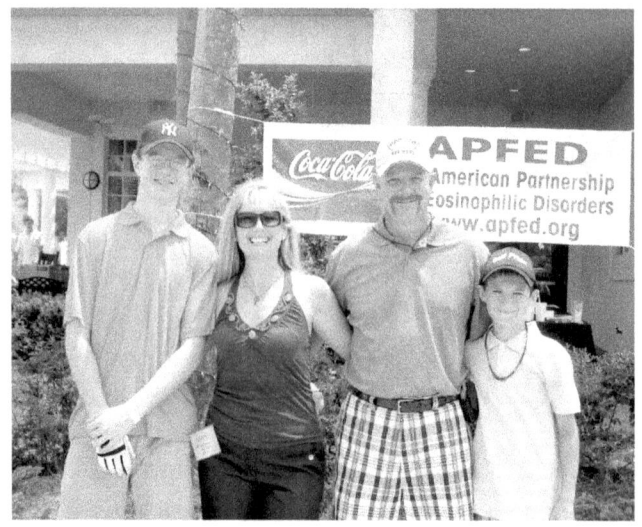

Walls family at the Remington Walls Golf Tournament to benefit Apfed, 2010

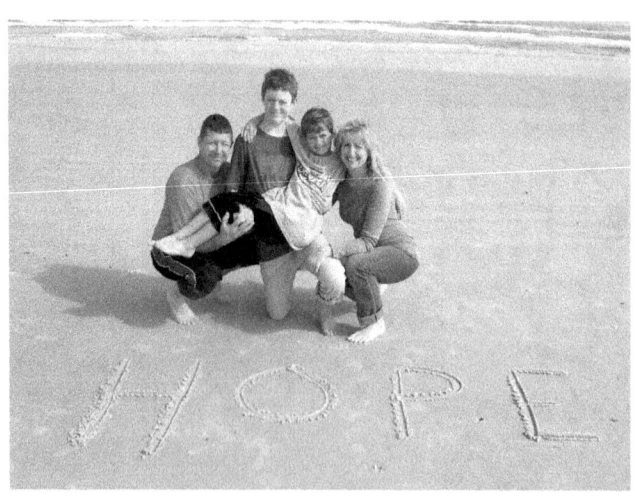

Walls family inspired by their family's word of HOPE

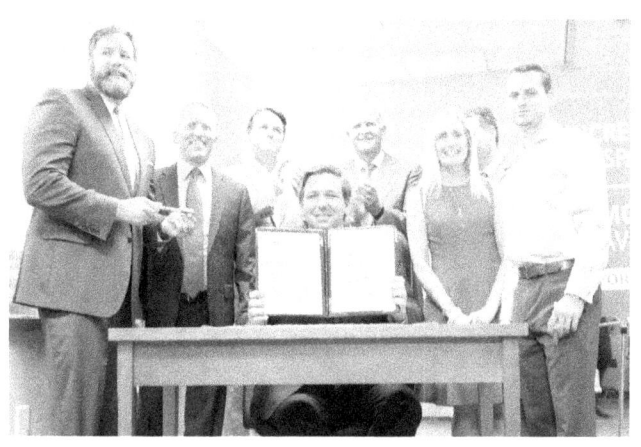

Governor Ron DeSantis signs CS/HB 1113 also known as the Patient Savings Act on June 12, 2019

www.ingramcontent.com/pod-product-compliance
Lightning Source LLC
Chambersburg PA
CBHW071457080526
44587CB00014B/2137